Lots of Candles, Plenty of Cake

Anna Quindlen is a novelist and journalist whose work has appeared on fiction, non-fiction, and self-help bestseller lists. Her book *A Short Guide to a Happy Life* has sold more than a million copies. While a columnist at *The New York Times*, she won the Pulitzer Prize and published two collections, *Living Out Loud* and *Thinking Out Loud*. Her *Newsweek* columns were collected in *Loud and Clear*. She is the author of six novels, *Object Lessons*, *One True Thing*, *Black and Blue*, *Blessings*, *Rise and Shine*, and *Every Last One*.

ALSO BY ANNA QUINDLEN

FICTION

Every Last One
Rise and Shine
Blessings
Black and Blue
One True Thing
Object Lessons

NON-FICTION

Good Dog. Stay
Being Perfect
Loud and Clear
A Short Guide to a Happy Life
How Reading Changed My Life
Thinking Out Loud
Living Out Loud

BOOKS FOR CHILDREN

Happily Ever After
The Tree That Came to Stay

Praise for *Lots of Candles, Plenty of Cake*

'Like having an older, wiser sister or favorite aunt over for a cup of tea, Quindlen's latest book is full of the counsel and ruminations many of us wish we could learn young...A graceful look at growing older from a wise and accomplished writer.'

Kirkus

'Even if you haven't been taping Anna Quindlen's *New York Times* and *Newsweek* columns to your fridge for two or three decades, *Lots of Candles, Plenty of Cake* will engage you with the easy familiarity of a cozy chat with a friend who knows you, warts and all, and still loves you. In this memoir, Quindlen again offers her keen observations of a well examined, well lived life...A laugh-out-loud book...*Lots of Candles, Plenty of Cake* renews and restores our zest for life.'

The Washington Independent Review of Books

'Having endeared herself to generations of women, beginning with her eminently distinctive and intuitively perceptive "Life in the 30s" column, Quindlen now brings her considered and accepted voice of reflection and evaluation to the challenges and opportunities that await...Quindlen will delight her steadfast readers with this pithy, get-real memoir.'

Booklist

'Wise and inspiring...Quindlen masterfully and beautifully sums up the best parts of aging: thoroughly knowing yourself, truly not caring what others think, and enjoying the confidence and courage that come with decades of practicing life and finding out, remarkably, it mostly turns out okay.'

Huffington Post

'Sublime...From facing an empty nest at home to facing wrinkles in the mirror, she writes incisively about her life now and what she owes to the generations of women who came before her...With this provocative, moving new book, Quindlen proves she may be at the midpoint of life, but she's at the top of her game.'

BookPage

'Classic Quindlen, at times witty, at times wise, and always of her time.'

The Miami Herald

'Serves up generous portions of her wise, commonsensical, irresistibly quotable take on life in the 50s – and beyond... What Nora Ephron does for body image and Anne Lamott for spiritual neuroses, Quindlen achieves on the home front.'

NPR

'In *Lots of Candles, Plenty of Cake*, Quindlen does what she does best. She calmly and carefully untangles the fine strands of a woman's life by examining her own, and lays them out cleanly for all to see, this time from the perspective of a woman in her 50s.'

Star Tribune (Minneapolis)

'Delightful, wise and witty...an empowering, uplifting read for women at any stage of their life's journey.'

Book Reporter

'Imparts an abiding curiosity and zest for life.'

The Boston Globe

'A book to savor.'

Richmond Times-Dispatch

Lots of Candles, Plenty of Cake

ANNA QUINDLEN

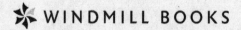 WINDMILL BOOKS

Published by Windmill Books 2013

4 6 8 10 9 7 5

Grateful acknowledgement is made to Faber and Faber Ltd for
permission to reprint lines from 'This Be The Verse' taken from
The Complete Poems © The Estate of Philip Larkin.

First published in the United States in 2012 by Random House,
an imprint of The Random House Publishing Group,
a division of Random House, Inc., New York

Windmill Books
The Random House Group Limited
20 Vauxhall Bridge Road, London SW1V 2SA

Addresses for companies within The Random House Group Limited can be found at:
www.randomhouse.co.uk/offices.htm

The Random House Group Limited Reg. No. 954009

www.randomhouse.co.uk

A CIP catalogue record for this book
is available from the British Library

ISBN 9780099559030

Book design by Susan Turner

Printed and bound by Clays Ltd, St Ives PLC

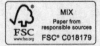

Penguin Random House is committed to a sustainable
future for our business, our readers and our planet.
This book is made from Forest Stewardship
Council® certified paper.

CONTENTS

Life in the Fifties

It's odd when I think of the arc of my life, from child to young woman to aging adult. First I was who I was. Then I didn't know who I was. Then I invented someone and became her. Then I began to like what I'd invented. And finally I was what I was again.

It turned out I wasn't alone in that particular progression.

I began to discover that twenty-five years ago, when I created a column about my own life for *The New York Times* called "Life in the 30's." The thirty-four-year-old mother of two little boys, I was shaky and unsure, wondering whether their stories of sibling rivalry and toilet training, my stories of household juggling and family accommodations, would have any resonance outside the walls of our home.

I got the answer to that question soon enough. From kitchens in Winnetka and Austin and Westport and Chevy Chase the messages arrived: You are writing my life. My sons do the same thing yours do. My friends offer the same solace. The moms in my playgroup have the same advice and issues. Sometimes people would suggest I must have been eavesdropping in their living rooms. Often they would report that they had put a particular column on their refrigerator. "Fridgeworthy," one woman said of a piece I wrote about lightning bugs. As I sat in front of my primitive computer, typing as fast as I could because I never knew when I would be interrupted by the appearance of the toddler in the home office or a howl from the baby from the floor below, I could imagine that fridge, a fridge like the one in my own kitchen, with its collection of *Sesame Street* magnets and blurry family photos, emergency phone contacts and preschool schedules.

"I feel like I'm not alone," some of those who wrote to me said, and that sentiment changed my life. That's what's so wonderful about reading, that books and poetry and essays make us feel as though we're connected, as though the thoughts and feelings we believe are singular and sometimes nutty are shared by others, that we are all more alike than different. It's the wonderful thing about writing, too. Sometimes I would think I was the only person alive concerned about some crazy cul-de-sac of human behavior. Then I would get the letters from readers and realize that that was not the case, that we were not alone, any of us.

Often we felt as though we were. We were living odd patchwork lives in those years because of an accident of timing. We were the daughters of women who had moved directly from their parents' homes to those of their husbands, gone right from high school to marriage and motherhood. But my friends and I had gone to college, entered the work world, under the rubric of the New Woman, suddenly able through vast changes in societal mores to use our abilities in the world and combine them with a domestic life at home. We were the heiresses to a women's movement that had broken the world wide open. But we were completely making it up as we went along, at work, at home, in our own minds, trying to be both our mothers and our fathers simultaneously. That wasn't easy.

One of the great unspoken effects of all this was a vast loneliness that went untouched because it went undiscussed. The women's movement had famously created consciousness-raising groups in which feminists discussed their grievances, but there was no corollary for those who had found so many of their wishes fulfilled and yet found this unfulfilling, exhausting, or even impossible. While the women of our mothers' generation felt constrained not to complain that no-wax floors and bridge parties were not exactly stimulating, we didn't want to admit that trying to balance a couple of challenging full-time jobs was kind of a stretch. We were all a little happy and a little crazy and a little sad and a little confused. And we all thought it was just us. That's what makes life so hard for women, that instead of thinking that this is the way things are, we always think it's the way *we* are.

My last "Life in the 30's" column began with a one-sentence birth announcement: "Her name is Maria"—the news that Quin and Chris now had a little sister and I was going to be too addled, with a newborn and two little boys, to write for a while. I moved on, and so did the readers. Our kids grew up and our marriages matured or, in some cases, imploded. We got promoted or didn't, stayed where we were planted or went somewhere else.

Time passed, almost imperceptibly. First we were so young and then we were so busy and then one day we awoke to discover that we were an age we once thought of as old. When I wrote about my life and discovered that it intersected with the lives of so many women like me, most of us were concerned with just managing to hold things together, managing to move from school drop-off to work assignments to making dinner to homework supervision to nodding off over the evening news, with the occasional truncated conversation thrown in, or not. We were trying to make it through each day, and then suddenly we looked around and realized the days were months, were years, and, almost magically and unconsciously, we had made it through a couple of decades.

Once again we were improvising: our grown kids still living at home or needing support, our aged parents requiring care. The most liberated generation of women in American history, raised on the notion that they could be much more than caregivers, became caregivers cubed. Because of longer life spans and different ways of living and working, once again we were pioneers. The year I was born, the average American lived to be sixty-eight; today that's closer to eighty. We've added a decade to our body clocks. But that extra time comes not at the end, when things are pretty much what they always were—physical degeneration, systematic loss, more of a look back than a look ahead; it comes now in the years between sixty and seventy, years that feel like an encore instead of a coda.

Many of us have come to a surprising conclusion about this moment in our lives. No, it's not that there are weird freckly spots on the back of our hands, although there are, or that construction guys don't make smutty comments as we pass, although they don't. It's that we've done a pretty good job of becoming ourselves, and that this is, in so many ways, the time of our lives. As Carly Simon once sang, "These are the good old days." Lots of candles, plenty of cake. I wouldn't be twenty-five again on a bet, or even forty. And when I say this to a group of women at lunch, everyone around the table nods. Many of us find ourselves exhilarated, galvanized, at the very least older and wiser.

The fridge looks different now. The college calendar, the kids' business cards, the number of Dad's cardiologist, the invitation to the bridal shower for the daughter of a friend, and a magnet that says YOU'RE NEVER TOO OLD . . . TO TRY SOMETHING

STUPID. I have that magnet. I have that fridge. Photographs of friends now gone, squiggle drawings by genius grandchildren—they wait in the wings. What comes next? Who knows? It's a long story, the story of our lives—the friends, the families, the men, the jobs, the mistakes we made and the ones we avoided, the tedium, the drama. Some things I took a long time to figure out, and others I'll never understand. All I can say for sure is that I want more.

To be continued.

PART I

The Laboratory of Life

*Life must be lived forward
but understood backward.*

—Søren Kierkegaard

Recently my twenty-two-year-old daughter asked me what message I would give to my own twenty-two-year-old self if I could travel back in time. I instantly had two responses, one helpful, one not. On the one hand, I would tell my younger self that she should stop listening to anyone who wanted to smack her down, that she was smart enough, resourceful and hardworking enough, pretty terrific in general. On the other hand, I would have to break the bad news: that she knew nothing, really, about anything that mattered. Nothing at all. Not a clue.

You don't know what you don't know when you're young. How could you? People who are older nod sagely and say you'll learn—about love, about marriage, about failing and falling down and getting up and trying to stagger on toward success, about work and children and what really matters, in general and to you. It's not, they'll say, what's on your business card, at a moment when you don't even have a business card. I recall hearing this message constantly when I was younger, and thinking that I was getting older as fast as I could. In retrospect this seems a bit of a shame as well as a vainglorious task. You're like a cake when you're young. You can't rush it or it will fall, or just turn out wrong. Rising takes patience, and heat.

It's nothing short of astonishing, all that we learn between the time we are born and the time we die. Of course most of the learning takes place not in a classroom or a library, but in the laboratory of our own lives. We can look back and identify moments—the friend's betrayal, the work advancement or failure, the wrong turn or the romantic misstep, the careless comment. But it's all a continuum that is clear only in hindsight, frequently when some of its lessons may not even be useful anymore.

Maybe that's why we give advice, when we're older, mostly to people who don't want to hear it. They can't hear it because it's in a different language, a language we learn over time, the language of experience cut with failure, triumph, and tedium. We finally understand childrearing when our children are grown. We look back on our work and know now how we would have altered plans and strategies, realize that some of what seemed inevitable at the time could have been altered, different. We understand ourselves, our lives, retrospectively.

There comes that moment when we finally know what matters and, perhaps more important, what doesn't, when we see that all the life lessons came not from what we had but from who we loved, and from the failures perhaps more than the successes.

I would tell my twenty-two-year-old self that what lasts are things so ordinary she may not even see them: family dinners, fair fights, phone calls, friends. But of course the young woman I once was cannot hear me, not just because of time and space but because of the language, and the lessons, she has yet to learn. It's a miracle: somehow over time she learned them all just the same, by trial and error.

Stuff

*Time is at once the most valuable and the most
perishable of all our possessions.*

—John Randolph,
colonial member of Congress

I have a lot of stuff. I bet you do, too. Sofas, settees, bureaus, bookshelves. Dishes, bowls, pottery, glass, candlesticks, serving trays, paperweights. Beds, chests, trunks, tables. Windsor chairs, club chairs, ladder-back chairs, folding chairs, wicker chairs. Lots and lots of chairs.

I have needlepoint pillows everywhere: camels, chickens, cats, houses, barns, libraries, roses, daisies, pansies. I needlepoint while I watch television. I have a vision of my children, after I'm gone, looking around and saying, "What are we going to do with all these pillows?" I don't mind. My best friend, Janet, has more pillows than I do, and more platters, too. Once I bought some plates and knew instantly that she would love them. "Where did you get those?" she asked, and I lied to her and then bought some for her birthday.

"Did she need more plates?" asked my husband, whose idea of need is different from my own.

In the city I have lots of stuff on the walls. Modern art, traditional art, landscapes, photographic prints. Eclectic. In the country I have samplers. THE BLESSING OF THE HOME IS CONTENTMENT. THIS IS OUR HOUSE / THE DOOR OPENS WIDE / AND WELCOMES YOU / TO ALL INSIDE. I have a large piece of framed embroidery that shows a woman with bobbed hair and an apron holding a tray with a tea service. A GOOD HOUSEWIFE MAKES A GOOD HOME, this one says. Lots of people who come to our house, knowing my politics, think it's ironic.

It's not ironic.

I didn't have all this stuff when I was young and single. None of us did. It was a big deal to have blinds and coffee mugs. Many of the guys I knew didn't; they'd tack a sheet over the bedroom window, drink from Styrofoam. My first apartment was pretty typical; I had a small uncomfortable sleeper sofa, a bentwood rocker, a coffee table that was actually a trunk—didn't everyone in 1976?—and a set of bookshelves. I was proud of those bookshelves. Many of my friends still used plastic egg crates, or plywood and cinder blocks.

In the bedroom I had a chest of drawers and a desk that was too low for an adult, at which I would hunch over my old manual Smith Corona typewriter, my knees contorted beneath. I had swapped the twin bed of my girlhood for a double bed, which children nowadays, raised on queen-size beds from seventh grade, the first generation of middle-class kids who trade down when they arrive in college dorms, can scarcely imagine. I was proud of that double bed. Many of my friends had futons.

That was more or less it. My stuff then would all fit in the back of one U-Haul, and not the big one, either. None of us used movers when we changed apartments, just called around and got a group together for pizza and beer and haulage. A lot of stuff wound up on the sidewalk for the sanitation truck.

But then we got married and we got carafes, chafing dishes, and china. We bought matching love seats for the living room in the row house that had once been a rooming house. ("Your grandfather worked hard all his life so his grandchildren wouldn't have to live in a place like this," my father said, sitting on the stoop, but he still lent us money for the renovation.) I trawled junk shops for oak furniture too old to be new but too young to be antique. I had a brief flirtation with Fiesta ware and Roseville pottery, never met a big old bowl or platter I couldn't love. When we were in Sicily for his sister's twentieth birthday and I halted, transfixed, before a window display of Italian pottery, our older son said, deadpan, "Mom, why don't you get one of those so you can put it on a little stand on a shelf somewhere?" I'd never really thought they'd noticed, much less passed judgment.

And that's not even counting the stuff in my closet. One day I peered inside and realized it looked like it belonged to someone with multiple personality disorder. The bohemian look, the sharp suits, the frilly dresses. Those days are behind me, and I finally know who and how I'm dressing. I'm dressing a person who has eighteen pairs of black pants and eleven pairs of black pumps. Of course, that number is illusory, since it includes the black pants I never felt looked great but purchased on sale, the pair that never seem to be the right length, and the two pairs that fit funny. Not too big or too small, just funny. Naturally there are two pairs of the shoes that I wear all the time, because they're comfortable, and one pair that I wear on occasion because they are great-looking and my toes don't go entirely numb for at least three hours.

I prefer not to dwell on the purses and the white T-shirts. You know, fashion magazines always say you can never have too many white T-shirts.

Yes, you can.

It wasn't always like this, was it? At some point in America, desire and need became untethered in our lives, and shopping became a competitive sport. I can't recall my mother spending much time spending, although of course she predated that black hole of consumption, the shopping website. It was generally agreed in our family that my grandmother Quindlen was a world-class shopper, and there was a much-repeated, often-embellished story about one of my aunts arriving early enough at a big sale to score a spot at the front of the line and still finding my grandmother already inside the store when she'd breached the doors. But there was always an object to the hunt: a Hitchcock chair, a pair of Naturalizer pumps. Sometimes I feel as though credit cards have helped us concentrate on quantity, not quality; the other day a financial adviser on TV said that if people were using cash for purchases, they tended to be much more abstemious. Plastic is magical, as though the bill will never come due.

I have too much plastic, too, in my wallet.

What do we notice when we drive down the highways of our adolescence and measure what's changed? We now have the big-box stores, the home emporiums, the fast-food places, certainly, but the weirdest addition is the thousands of storage facilities that loom, bunkerlike, windowless. When we were kids, storage was the basement and attic, a broken chair, an army trunk. Today we rent facilities for the stuff we're not currently using, probably will never use again.

Statisticians say our houses are almost twice as large, on average, as they were forty years ago. So much stuff, rotating rooms of it: cribs, big-boy beds, changing tables, desks, new linens, new window treatments, new rugs. When my kids got their own places, they went shopping in the junk shops in the top and bottom stories of our own homes. My husband says that when you go to their apartments it's like a walk down Memory Lane, that little table we never really found a place for, the coffee mugs that take both of us right back to the era when there was scarcely time for coffee because someone always needed a glass of milk or a story read. "Take more!" I kept saying, but they demurred, not wanting to seem greedy. The odd frying pan, the chipped bowls. Quin cleans, Christopher cooks. Chris called one night and asked how to drain spaghetti if you don't have one of those things with the holes in it. Next time he came over I gave him one of my four colanders. Or maybe it's five. I like the old enameled ones.

The nicest thing you can say to me about my home is that it's homey, and people say it all the time. I like it. And at a certain point, I can't say when, I realized I didn't really give a damn about any of it. If there were a fire, what would I save? We all used to say it was the photo albums, but with digital photography we all have our photographs on our computers, on Facebook, in emails to our families and friends. My cookbooks are well thumbed, but I know the best recipes by heart now, and the bad recipes I've either discarded or adapted.

I can't even say I would reach for the wedding album; it seems so long ago, and so many of our friends didn't come into our lives until afterward. There's a porcelain bird I gave my mother the Christmas before she died, which she owned for less than a month, that I've wrapped carefully in tissue and taken with me from the small apartment to the bigger apartment to the brownstone to the nicer brownstone. There are the letters my kids write each year to Santa Claus, even now that they no longer watch me seal them in envelopes and address them to S. Claus, North Pole, 99705 (which is really the zip code of North Pole, Alaska, not the real North Pole), even now that my daughter has learned to write to Santa online and to insert a web link so you can click on the letter to Santa and go directly to the dress she wants from Saks in the correct size and color. There's the mink coat my husband gave me when our first child was born, which I haven't worn for years because our kids are bothered by fur but which I treasure because it made me feel prosperous, elegant, and wifelike for perhaps the first time.

If there were a fire I'd probably just grab a few old pictures and the Labradors. I'd be wearing the watch and the rings my husband gave me for the big birthdays. I haven't removed my wedding ring since the day he put it on me and the priest blessed it. I'd miss the rest, but I wouldn't mourn it. Except for the Christmas ornaments, I guess. My entire family is pretty attached to the Christmas ornaments.

It could be that I'm fooling myself about all this, the way I tell myself that if I didn't have so much on my plate I would spend six months living in London or Virgin Gorda when the truth is that if I didn't have so much on my plate I would watch more old movies and forward lots of stupid Internet jokes to my children. It's not that I want to trade the old stuff for new stuff. Every time I try that, I wind up re-creating what I already have; I swear that I'm finally going to have furnishings that are soft and serene, cream and ecru, and before you know it everything's red again. Besides, I'm always mesmerized by those women who completely redecorate. The room was blue and yellow with overstuffed sofas and distressed pine, and then one day it's off-white and celery (which is what shelter magazines call pale green) with low chaises and glass tables. My house is not like that; no clean sweeps for me. The brass bed in Christopher's old room is the one Gerry and I slept in when we were first married. The mahogany bowfront chest under the windows in the den is part of what used to be called a bedroom suite that belonged to my parents. The furniture in the country house mainly came with it; I still have the engraved stationery of Mrs. Frederick W. Trumpbour in one of the cubbyholes in the cherry drop-front desk. The china cabinet in the New York City living room I bought for twenty-five dollars at a legendary flea market in Englishtown, New Jersey, and drove through the Holland Tunnel with its mahogany pediment jutting from the back of the car. It's never closed that well, but still! Twenty-five dollars!

Obviously I don't need stuff to remind me of my own life if I can remember how much I paid for a not-quite antique on a Saturday morning thirty-five years ago. I'm not certain I need the stuff anymore at all, except maybe my collection of nun paraphernalia, a gift from Christopher that I intend to leave to the weirdest of his children. The doctor checks my height every time I have a physical, and I'm a little shirty about it, bound and determined that I will stand tall, that my bones are brilliant, that I will not shrink. But somehow I feel a pronounced urge now to shrink my surroundings, to stick to just a few comfortable rooms, to have less instead of more. I feel as though I am at the peak of a progression, and from here I should follow another gentle downward slope: smaller, tighter, cleaner, simpler. No clutter. Less stuff. I'm not sure why this is the case. Maybe it's because I now feel I know the truth about possessions, that they mean or prove or solve nothing. Stuff is not salvation.

My friend Susan is my role model in this. She and her husband and their three boys have somehow forgone the entire era of crazed consumerism. When they have stuff, it has a purpose, a point; when they acquire something, it has resonance and meaning, whether it's a dirt bike or a new television. They get honey from their bees, eggs from their chickens, venison the way you do out in the country, where hunting trumps the supermarket. Susan and her many sisters have swap meets each year in which they shop around among one another's clothing. And on Christmas several years ago her youngest, Willem, then a very little boy, was permitted, in his family's fashion, to open one gift on Christmas Eve. The next morning, when he saw his stack of presents under the tree, he said, "But I already have one."

Do I need to mention that they are a happy family?

I'm not sure I could have seen that when I was younger. I

somehow believed that if you had matching side chairs and a sofa that harmonized and some beautiful lamps to light them all and some occasional tables with family photographs in frames scattered around them that you would have a home, that visual harmony and elegance promoted happiness. I fooled myself into thinking that *House Beautiful* should be subtitled *Life Wonderful*. I don't know why I thought this, since the home in which I grew up as the oldest of five was always pretty topsy-turvy, the dining room table turned into a fort with blankets, the *chunk-chunk* of someone jumping on the bed upstairs. I should have learned my lesson years ago, when we went to the grandest wedding imaginable and the couple divorced within a few years, or when we went to dinner at an apartment on Fifth Avenue that was so beautiful and bright it was hard to know where to look and our host and hostess spent the entire evening sniping at each other. Maybe it took me a long time to get over the afternoon when I dropped one of my mother's Royal Doulton figurines and she burst into tears. She had so few nice things, so few things that weren't grubby with fingerprints or sticky with jelly.

But there's so much responsibility to stuff. I should have realized that at that moment, seeing the little dancing Doulton woman in Regency garb headless on the kitchen floor. Stuff needs to be dusted and insured and willed to someone without hurting someone else's feelings. (Those of you with one daughter and two sons surely know the look of incredulous horror that accompanies the suggestion that your jewelry will be divided three ways. "But the boys' wives won't even really be your family!" your daughter shrieks.) You have a nice chair, and then one day the fabric is in tatters and it all begins: swatches, furniture trucks, upholsterers, weeks and weeks of waiting, weeks and weeks of peering at it afterward and wondering if you've made a mistake.

And what does any of this have to do with real life? Real life is relaxed, as I was after the Corian countertop had been in for a year or two and I stopped attacking the tiny nicks from the knives with fine sandpaper while my husband made himself scarce, afraid he'd be held responsible.

Here's what it comes down to, really: there is now so much stuff in my head, so many years, so many memories, that it's taken the place of primacy away from the things in the bedrooms, on the porch. My doctor says that, contrary to conventional wisdom, she doesn't believe our memories flag because of a drop in estrogen but because of how crowded it is in the drawers of our minds. "We women today have more on the hard disc than any women at any time in history," she says. Between the stuff at work and the stuff at home, the appointments and the news and the gossip and the rest, the past and the present and the plans for the future, the filing cabinets in our heads are not only full, they're overflowing.

Sometimes they appear to be full of random stuff anyhow, the name of the actress who played Scarlett's sister in *Gone with the Wind* (Evelyn Keyes) and the area code for the city where I went to convent school (314) instead of the name of the restaurant where I'm supposed to be meeting a friend for lunch in an hour or the location of my keys. My mother just had to keep the home stuff straight, my father what was going on at work. But women today need to keep track of both, along with what's going on in the world and what's going on with the kids. The birthday party, the husband's mother, the friend's book party, the work deadlines, the grocery shopping, the bills. Stuff stuff stuff stuff.

Maybe my overstuffed brain makes me want to have barer surroundings, more space, to shuck the Ali Baba cave of my own existence. Everything that was once the right size for five people is too big for two. Lots of people tell me to wait awhile and I can put my grandchildren in their parents' old rooms when they come to stay. I wonder what they'll find in the backs of the closets and the bottoms of the drawers. Oooh, Dad, rolling papers and dirty magazines.

One day I saw a modular house in the newspaper. It was built of metal and glass in some Scandinavian country (of course) and sent here by freighter boat, complete with some Scandinavians to assemble it on-site for the buyer. A big living room, a tiny kitchenette, a small bathroom and bedroom. We could clear a space in the woods across the road from our big old house, furnish it with a few modern pieces. Perfection.

"I already have a house," my husband said flatly when I was finished rhapsodizing.

This is what he says each time I want to change where and how we live: I already have a house. My husband doesn't care about stuff. Here's what he needs: A comfortable chair in which to read and watch TV. Sharp knives. A bottle opener. A pillow that, per the Goldilocks story, is neither too soft nor too hard. When he breaks a bowl while he's doing the dinner dishes, he always gets a terrible look on his face, but it's not because he is thinking, imported Italian Deruta in the Orvieto pattern. He always says, "I'm so sorry. I know you really liked this one." He's said it a dozen times.

It's Thoreau who wrote about this most indelibly and directly: "Simplify, simplify." (He also said, "It is a great art to saunter," which I think of from time to time when I walk down the street at a double-time city clip.) Tocqueville was more expansive: "Americans cleave to the things of the world as if assured they will never die. They clutch everything but hold nothing fast, and so lose grip as they hurry after some new delight."

And then there's Bob Quindlen, my father, who some years ago started to divest, sending and bringing me things, things that were either part of the past or forgotten gifts: framed photographs of his grandchildren, an old pitcher in the shape of a pig that had been in my mother's kitchen, an antique butter press designed to emboss the butter with the letter Q, which, believe me, is a rare alphabetical find. It still has the gift card I placed inside it years ago, so faded that I can read only the first few lines, which begin, "This has no practical use in the 20th century." I was a little miffed that my father had given it back to me; now I'm figuring exactly when I should give it to our elder son, whose first name is the same as my last and who knows from experience how hard it is to find anything with a Q on it.

The sampler I like best is over the stove, where I spend a lot of my time, poaching eggs, poking a fork into the pot roast. I've committed its words to memory: WORK LIKE YOU DON'T NEED THE MONEY. LOVE LIKE YOU'VE NEVER BEEN HURT. DANCE LIKE NO ONE'S LOOKING. It could go up in flames with all the rest. I don't need stuff to remind me of that. That's a lesson I learned over time, when I wasn't distracted by acquisition. When I fall back into the old ways, I remember Willem saying on Christmas morning, "But I already have one." That's my new mantra, and it applies to almost everything.

Next of Kin

One August evening in 1978 my husband got a wonky serving at the Clam Shack and was so ill by 2:00 A.M. that I woke our friend David to drive him to Nantucket Cottage Hospital. A nurse took Gerry away looking like what an English acquaintance once called "death eating a cracker," and David and I sat slumped sleepily, silent, in the empty waiting room. The only magazines were *Highlights for Children* and *Sports Illustrated.* The nurse returned with a clipboard and said, "Are either of you related to him?" and we both shook our heads until David gave me a searching look. "Oh, oh, I'm his wife," I said, as though "wife" was a relationship somewhere south of third cousin once removed.

Related to him: it wasn't what I'd imagined when I slid down the aisle of the shrine of St. Joseph in a lace gown with bishop sleeves that I found at Bergdorf's. (For the record, if I had it to do over again it's still the dress I'd wear.) I dated a guy; I fell in love with a guy. And I figured I was going to date him and be in love with him as long as we both shall live. You dream yourself a life out of bits of fantasy and imaginings, like cotton candy, pink and mostly air. And then you have an actual life that has almost nothing to do with the cotton candy one. I didn't really think about the fact that we would be each other's next of kin. I didn't think about being kin at all. In some ways "kin" is the antithesis of "boyfriend." It took me almost a year to call him "my husband" with any regularity. On our second date I told him that I wouldn't change my surname if I ever married. "I don't think you have to worry about that," he said.

For our twenty-fifth anniversary a group of our friends gave us a tree. It sure has grown. It's a model of what a tree should be, the kind of thing a seven-year-old girl draws, a nice straight crayon-brown trunk with an oval of green leaves and a ring of flowers around it. (Seven-year-old boys draw stick figures and dinosaurs that look like lumpy dogs. I'm sorry, but it's true.)

"Oh, that's a Bradford pear," said the arborist who came to look at the finicky trees, the ones that get fungus and big long-fingered dead limbs. "It's almost a weed, it grows so easily."

Bad metaphor for marriage, although that's not what you think when you're young and it's your first time out. If you're getting married for the right reasons, because this guy keeps cracking you up and he has a great grin and he never says "How much money can you really make as a writer?" you think being married is going to be like a Bradford pear tree, green and happy, flowering and spreading. If you looked down the long corridor of life and imagined the two of you at forty driving a kid to the emergency room with blood on the backseat, or thought about what it would be like when you were fifty-five and one of you got pink-slipped, or conjured the new guy at your office who tells you he thinks you have great eyes or the young woman at his who hangs on every word he says at the Friday evening bar breaks, you'd begin to realize that it's a different kind of tree altogether. But we don't do that. We can't. The best we can do is look at the long marriages of others. If they're good, or seem good, we tell ourselves that's how we'll be. If they're bad, it's their own fault.

I don't want to throw in my lot with the marriage-is-hard-work crowd, the ones who suggest you see a couples counselor before you send out the invitations, who seem to support the entire advice-book industry. I was never one of those women who tell you that their spouse is their best friend, that they're always on the same page. I feel like you're ahead of the game if you're even in the same book.

Part of the problem, obviously, is that we've gotten as greedy about marriage as we have about so much else. And because we are so invested in youthful behavior, we have youthful illusions abetted by a culture that insists that the conversation, libido, interaction, attraction, and relationship of two people who have been together for forty years should be more or less like that of two people who have been together for only a few months. This makes no sense, nor should it. What if I said that I still wrote in much the same way, about most of the same things, as I did when I was eighteen? What if my husband had developed no new techniques or strategies for trying a case after decades as a trial lawyer? That wouldn't be seen as reassuring or normative but as terrible.

Perspective is a good thing. You can't take the long view without it. And for an enduring marriage today, the long view is what's required. In 1900, one estimate has it, the average marriage lasted twenty-three years. Today, unless divorce or untimely death intervenes, the average marriage can be expected to last more than twice that long. In fact, that's part of the explanation for the boom in late-in-life divorces between people who have been together for decades. With longer life expectancies, a woman in her sixties who is unhappily attached is looking at another twenty years and decides to say "No way" despite the shock and dismay of family and friends. Monogamy sometimes seems designed for a time when life was shorter and expectations lower. When I was a child and people would ask my father how long he and my mother had been married, he would sometimes reply, "She was at my First Communion." He seemed to find this absolutely hilarious, while I always found it puzzling. But I am married to a man I met my freshman year in college, and sometimes I look across the dinner table at him and think, "He was at my First Communion."

When I first married, I expected my husband to be all things: sex object, professional sounding board, partner in parenting, constant companion. I pretended interest in everything he was interested in, and eventually some of them even interested me, like the New Deal and the New York Yankees. (I will never get on board with NASCAR.) The things I didn't expect him to be were the ones that, in centuries past, had given the shape of a contract to matrimony, chief among them the transaction in which he made the money and I made the home. We had a partnership, all in all. Many of us blithely assumed this was a very good deal for everyone involved. The mental image of one of us wearing an apron and the other a suit, what the TV shows of our childhoods might have called the "Honey, I'm home" effect, seemed to imply an arid and empty existence. Poor her, with nothing to think about but the living room drapes and the tuna casserole. Poor him, with the weight of the world on his shoulders. Poor them, with little in common.

It turned out that some of this was hooey. Lots of those old-fashioned marriages were happy ones, in part because no one expected to look over and see their best friend in the adjoining twin bed. (Twin beds, we thought to ourselves!) And it turned out that some of the terms of the new egalitarian partnerships were not that great for those involved. It was difficult to grow up with one set of expectations and responsibilities, then to live through a societal bait-and-switch the likes of which no generation of men and women had ever seen before. My father has said from time to time that he wonders whether his marriage to my mother, the most domestic of spouses, could have survived the women's movement and perhaps her determination to have a different sort of life. Once on a train I heard an older couple arguing heatedly and after a minute or two realized that the fight was about his habit of referring to the money he gave her each week as an allowance. "I am not a child, John," she said, and nothing he could say jollied her out of a silence that hung over their two seats like a cloud until they disembarked in Baltimore.

My husband and I have together created three children, but we have separate finances, and that's the way I like it. It's not because, as Abigail Adams once wrote in her habitual harsh fashion, "All men would be tyrants if they could." I'm just realistic: we're not two hearts that beat as one. (In any marriage I've ever known in which two hearts beat as one, the one is his. Here's to you, Abigail Adams.) Instead, we're two strong-minded people who have divergent talents and habits. Gerry loves the fall and hates the heat; I prefer summer and I am sanguine about humidity. He's not the least bit interested in celebrity gossip; it's a really bad habit, and I'm sticking with it. He balances his checkbook, and I'm pretty sure that everything will come out okay at the end of the month. He believes in washing dishes by hand, and I'm a dishwasher zealot. When we first met I venerated the Beatles, he the Rolling Stones; I have to admit that over the years he's brought me closer to Mick, not a bad place to be.

I used to joke that Gerry had never been known to apply heat to food, but since he started making oatmeal for both of us on winter mornings I've had to give up that allegedly humorous observation. He says he doesn't cook because he doesn't have to, given that I'm so good at it. That's the kind of compliment you don't even recognize as a compliment after a couple of decades together unless you take the time to hold it up to the light and let the sun shine through it.

Like bumper cars, each of us moves the other into unfamiliar territory a bit. Or not. As the comedian Rita Rudner says, "It's great to find that one special person you want to annoy for the rest of your life." We're part of a mixed marriage: he's male, I'm female. It's not personal, it's gender-based, like the conversations that go like this:

What did we decide about that dinner party the HooHas invited us to?

We talked about that the other night.

We did?

Yes.

What did we decide?

Lord, all this has driven me nuts over the years. You never listen to me. You always forget. You never help. You always say that. You never do that. Petty grievances in marriage are like hothouse tomatoes: they get way bigger than they ought to, and they bear little resemblance to the real thing. A couple of years ago I saw a cartoon in *The New Yorker* in which, at the dinner table, wife says to husband, "Pass the salt, pass the salt—what am I, your slave?"

The term "soul mate"—which, I'm proud to say, I have never once used until now—suggests two people who have everything in common. But our gender, with all the differences it implies, divides us. That has its advantages: most of the men I know scarcely remember petty slights, while I nurse mine like kittens. My husband seems naturally inclined to cede certain areas of our family life to me. I can decorate any way I want as long as the big chair faces the flat-screen TV, with a table next to it for beer and cashews. And that's just fine. Frankly, I don't want a husband who knows what toile is. The one piece of furniture in whose purchase my husband actually participated was our first couch. It was so long ago that the couch cost a thousand dollars, so whenever I buy anything new and he asks how much it cost—an armoire, an Oriental rug, a six-burner gas stove that came in at around the same price as my first car—I say a thousand dollars. A safety net of small white lies can be the bedrock of a successful marriage. You wouldn't believe how cheaply I can do a kitchen renovation. Neither would any kitchen renovator, including the one I actually used.

If you're an inveterate reader you can't help noticing that most great art evades all of this completely. Jane Austen wrote some of the finest books in the history of literature, but the unmarried novelist draws the blinds on every one of her protagonists once the vows have been uttered. (Only the secondary characters have long unions, and too often they are either stupid women and the men who married them for their now-faded beauty, or stupid men and the women who married them for their considerable fortunes.) Do the fireworks between Mr. Darcy and Elizabeth Bennet that make *Pride and Prejudice* so incandescent result, ten years out, in slammed doors and sullen silences? We will never know, although the thought seems terrible. George and Martha tear at each other onstage in *Who's Afraid of Virginia Woolf,* while Romeo and Juliet get a couple of good nights as teenagers, then die.

The trouble is that writing about a long and successful marriage is a little like writing about the newspaper business, which, not coincidentally, is also a line of work that doesn't appear much in novels. There are signal moments, bursts of excitement, times of dislocation and distress, buried within long stretches of uneventful everyday. And over time those long stretches create something that is challenging to illustrate in movies or plays or books. They create a blanket of real life, woven day by day until the thing is all of a piece. "There is no substitute for the comfort supplied by the utterly taken-for-granted relationship," Iris Murdoch wrote.

That's what I didn't understand when I married all those years ago. My vows were from Walt Whitman: "Camerado, I give you my hand. I give you my love more precious than money, I give you myself before preaching or law. Will you give me yourself? Will you come travel with me? Shall we stick by each other as long as we live?" Okay, cut me a break: I was young, romantic, and hyperliterary. Mostly young. But I'm proud that I chose words that are as redolent of a long journey as they are of romantic love, because that's ultimately what you wind up with, a journey that includes shared experience, setbacks, challenges, knowledge, and many many things that make you crazy as well as some things that make you happy. If a marriage is to endure over time, it has to be because both people within it have tacitly acknowledged something that young lovers might find preposterous: it's bigger, and more important, than both of us. It's love, sure, and inside jokes and conversational shorthand. But it's also families, friends, traditions, landmarks, knowledge, history. It's children, children whose parents' marriage is bedrock for them even if they're not children anymore. Perhaps especially if they're not children anymore.

One night years ago we were having dinner with old friends who had young children, and I mocked the notion of staying together for the sake of the kids. The woman leaned across the table and hissed at me fiercely, "That's a good reason to stay together." When I had children of my own I knew what she meant: not that children required tolerance of a terrible union, but that blowing up their world demanded a particularly searching look at your rationale for doing so.

This is not a brief against divorce. I've known people so ill-matched that even at their weddings we figured they were on borrowed time. I've known couples who, apart, were more generous and supportive of each other than they ever managed to be in tandem. And any number of my friends have had what I think of as starter marriages, an early childless union that was like a sunspot that once darkened their lives and was effortlessly lasered off. It's like my dad always told me about making pancakes: the first one just greases the grill and should be flipped right into the trash.

But I've also known couples who refused to break under weight that I assumed was crushing, couples who have weathered infidelity and tragedy and reversals of fortune. One of my friends, a psychologist, told me that the greatest determinant of whether a couple stays married is their determination to stay married; on the surface it sounded like a tautology, but the more I thought about it, the more sense it made to me.

Everyone thinks they know what they'd do in all these situations, especially if they've never been in them themselves. But it's certain that no one actually knows what goes on in a marriage except the two people involved, and often not even them. One of the most popular parlor games of my lifetime has been deconstructing the marriage of Bill and Hillary Clinton, the former president and the former First Lady, senator, presidential candidate, and secretary of state. Their imminent divorce has been predicted more often than the end of the world, and their continued union is explained by the cognoscenti in terms of political ambition. No one seems willing to allow that after all this time together, there may be something in their marriage for both of them, something deep and lasting and ultimately inexplicable. Maybe their marriage is flawed and fractured, and maybe it works for them. Or maybe they know what a divorced friend of mine admitted once, saying she had been too quick to end a union that was not wonderful but not terrible: "You think divorce is going to solve the problem, but it just creates a different set of problems." As the actor Jeff Bridges said when asked the secret of staying married in Hollywood, "Don't get divorced."

One day in the barbershop I heard a bunch of guys mocking

a young man who'd just left the shop. "Yeah, he'll find out after he's married," one snickered about the kid's moony attitude toward his girlfriend. All the others laughed, and various ball-and-chain comments followed. The thing to remember is that every one of those guys was married, and had been for a long time. In fact the barber himself spoke fondly, even fulsomely, to his wife during a phone call at some point in the middle of their marriage mockery. It made me wonder if our attitudes toward marriage are, in the last analysis, like what Winston Churchill once said of democracy: it's the worst system except for all the others.

Sometimes I tell my children—well, actually, frequently I tell my children—that the single most important decision they will make is not where to live, or what to do for a living, it's who they will marry. Part of this is the grandchild factor; I want mine to have two great parents if at all possible. But part is because the span of their years will be so marked by the life they build, day by day, in tandem with another. I fell for Gerry Krovatin when I was young and foolish because he looked great in a sports jacket, because he was a terrific dancer, because he was cool and smart and knew things I didn't, which I scarcely thought possible. He is focused, diligent, and funny; I am distractible, peripatetic, sometimes overly earnest. He's the first to criticize me privately and the first to defend me publicly. He has my back, and he always has. That's not romantic, and it's not lyrical, and it's not at all what I expected when I thought I would never want to spend a night without him. (Today I like a good solo business trip with trash TV and a room service breakfast as much as the next long-married woman.) But at this stage in my life, I'm not interested in being with people who don't have my back. All those I'm-just-telling-you-for-your-own-good types I knew when I was younger? Gone. There's a tight circle of backers who remain, and he's the backer-in-chief. He's mainly Irish, which means loyalty is somewhere between a physical reflex and a neurological response. He holds a grudge against anyone who does me wrong. He may not remember our social schedule or the names of some of our kids' friends, but he never forgets who wrote the bad review of my last book. And woe betide that individual if they ever meet him at a cocktail party. I like that in a man. Actually, I love that in a man.

Girlfriends

Ask any woman how she makes it through the day, and she may mention her calendar, her to-do lists, her baby-sitter. She may say that she's learned to let unnecessary tasks ride, that she no longer worries too much about home-cooked meals or clean countertops, that her go-to outfit of black pants and colored jacket is always waiting at the front of the closet, that she gets her reading done by listening to audiobooks in the car and sends email messages from her phone while she's having her hair cut.

But if you push her on how she really makes it through her day, or, more important, her months and years, how she stays steady when things get rocky, who she calls when the doctor says "I'd like to run a few more tests" or when her son moves in with the girl she's never much liked or trusted, she won't mention any of those things. She will mention her girlfriends. The older we get, the more we understand that the women who know and love us—and love us despite what they know about us—are the joists that hold up the house of our existence. Everything depends on them.

I'm not sure I would have said that at an earlier time of my life. To be a good friend and to appreciate the value of friendship requires honesty and concentration. It took a long time for the two to come together for me as an adult.

When I think back, I realize that in my own life there was a girlfriend interregnum, a time during which I lost the knack for, the connection to, but never the need for close female friends. I remember my early college reunions, how there was the crackle of jockeying in the air: who had a good job, a good husband, a good family, a good life, who was accomplished and who was a sellout and was there a difference? Who looked good, better, different, the same? I remember the later reunions, how enjoyable they were, surrounded by smart women who had become what theorists call "the integrated self," full of contradictions and compromises but at peace with both. Perhaps only when we've made our peace with our own selves can we really be the kind of friends who listen, advise, but don't judge, or not too harshly. My friends now are more cheerleader than critic. They are as essential to my life as my work or my home, a kind of freely chosen family, connected by ties of affinity instead of ties of blood.

This has come full circle for me since I was a child. When I was very young and life was uncomplicated, my girlfriends were the center of my existence. At the requisite time we became obsessed with boys, but when the boys actually materialized we went silent, afraid of saying too much, saying something wrong, seeming to be something we couldn't even put into words. (Smart? Strong? Perhaps I'm just projecting onto the past based on the present.) I had guy friends, and I still do, but it's not the same: easier in some ways, less emotional and fraught, but less profound, too. "If something bad happens, I go to my women friends for advice and my male friends for distraction," says my daughter.

When I was young it was when the boys weren't around that the conversations swirled, lying on my living room rug listening to 45s, staring into the dark at sleepovers. One of the big events in our neighborhood was the Bonner fair, a carnival at the local Catholic high school to which, when we were a certain age, a boy would invite us on what, in the broadest possible sense, might be called a date. Here was the great thing about the Bonner fair: talking about it for weeks in advance with your friends, planning what you were going to wear (something called an Ann-Margret blouse in a red bandanna print with ruffles that erupted at midbust, or would have if I'd actually been in possession of a bust at that time), getting dressed together, meeting up with the boys, talking about it afterward for weeks. The event itself was a blur of adrenaline and self-consciousness and, in my case, given how I feel about amusement park rides, nausea.

I spent two years of high school in a boarding school from which I was expelled; the school is no more but I'm still here, and I say that without jubilation since I was very happy there. It was a girls' school and so female friendship was more than ever pivotal, although it was there that I first began to realize that there were women who didn't like other women, who thought of them as poor substitutes until some guy came along. I also learned that, like marriages, many friendships are between people who are quite different and who fill in the unoccupied spaces in each other's characters. Ergo, Angie, who got nabbed sneaking out at night along with me. I was mouthy and combative, and the nuns assumed I had cooked the whole adventure up, so I got the heave-ho. Angie was—still is—good, kind, and sweet-tempered, and she went on to be the school's May Queen, to no one's surprise, including my own. For years I thought this was unfair, but now I think it was exactly as it ought to have been, especially once I took mouthy and combative out into the great world and found that there it worked better for me than it had in convent school.

It would be easy to say that the friendship drought that began after I was kicked out of Mount de Chantal Visitation Academy was a function of moving from the cloistered convent to a coeducational public high school, and there's probably some truth in that. There are endless studies that show that single-sex education, especially for girls, reinforces strength and diminishes the stranglehold of stereotypes, that it may lead girls toward everything from the study of mathematics to the pursuit of the Ph.D. I've realized that my attachment to girlfriends, the primacy of that bond, began to fray and disappear at the same time I decided I was no good at math. Coincidence? I don't think so. Feminist theory has it that girls tamp down their authentic selves after they reach puberty and don't really recover them until years later; when we turn away from who we are, we turn away from others like ourselves as well.

Returning to a single-sex environment in college, at Barnard, would seem to have been the antidote, and in some ways it was. It was a place that valued those qualities that adolescent social intercourse, not to mention the nuns at convent school, had not: opinions, opposition, argument, innovation. My time there dovetailed with the beginning of the second wave of feminism and the last gasp of the student struggles of the sixties, and a certain woman-warrior culture prevailed. It was the making of me as a human being, but it did not lead to an immediate resurgence of my friendship gene. The atmosphere was competitive and balkanized: the premeds, the radical feminists, the prospective writers. It should have been a safe place to be authentic, but I'm not certain many of us were. We'd merely taken out the part of the self that hadn't been safe to air in a more homogenized world and made her all in all, gone from the thesis of the compliant good girl to the antithesis of the self-possessed individualist.

Maybe that's what happens to all of us, why friendship ebbs and flows in many of our lives. That kind of connection to another human being is both soothing and scary, at once threatening and essential, because it reflects the tension in all of our lives between individuality and community. It's when we are young that we want to make certain the world understands we are absolutely and utterly distinct—it's why we mess around with the spelling of our names, wear strange clothes, streak our hair, get in trouble. When I was sixteen I was too busy telegraphing the fact that I was unique to want to embrace the notion of commonality. True friendship assumes a level playing field—no one is up, no one down, no one the queen bee or the drone. But young women often try to establish themselves as individuals by defining themselves in opposition to other women, which lends itself to exactly that kind of hierarchy and competition. The queen bee in the middle school classroom doesn't really have friends, she has followers. If the teenage girl had an ancestral crest, its motto would be "I am not you."

As we grow older the mythology has it that female friendships falter because we compete, for everything from the alpha job to the alpha male, but I didn't find that to be true. What I did find was that a frantic existence left too little time for friendship as it ought to be configured, deep and consistent. For decades I was focused on my work, my kids, my routine. I couldn't get out of my own head, much less my own house. The friends I made then were friends of proximity, other mothers on the playground, women whose husbands were friends of my husband. Some were office friends at a time when there were few women in the newsroom, and it was in the bathroom stall that I suppressed rage or tears. Some were political activists whose causes intersected with my writing and my inclinations. Those friendships that stuck were the ones in which one area overlapped with another, the fellow reporters who had children at the same time as I did, the playground moms whose husbands became friends with my husband. But when the proximity faded, some of those friendships did, too. There's an apt quote from Virginia Woolf: "I have lost friends, some by death, others through sheer inability to cross the street."

As we grow older we weed out our friendship circles the way we do our closets. Most women have a story about the friend who truly wasn't, whose calls and visits left her feeling dreadful, the friend who dined out on other women's shortcomings and mistakes. There are the friends that our spouses cannot bear, with whom we have lunch but rarely dinner, or the friend who drops us when someone better comes along. There are women who have serial best friends and those who stick with a childhood friend long past the time when they have anything in common except the memory of slumber parties and a mulish, uncompromising, enduring affection.

Sometimes I will see a photo of an actress in an unflattering dress or a blouse too young for her or a heavy-handed makeup job, and I mutter, "She must not have any girlfriends." We trust our friends to tell us what we need to know, and to shield us from what we don't need to discover, and to have the wisdom to know the difference. Real friends offer both hard truths and soft landings and realize that it's sometimes more important to be nice than to be honest. That, too, is knowledge that often comes only with age. Henry James wasn't exactly a warm fuzzy, so I think it's significant that even he once said, "Three things in human life are important: the first is to be kind, the second is to be kind, and the third is to be kind."

This is how the days begin for me now: I rise at 6:00 A.M., which would have been as improbable to my young self, who could roll over and go back to sleep with unconsidered ease, as would those evenings when I think idly, Is nine-thirty too early to go to bed? (No.) I go down to the kitchen, make enough coffee for several people even though I am the only one who drinks it, make the same breakfast every morning, either Greek yogurt with a little granola blended in or whole-grain bread with almond butter. Again, I can feel my younger self looking over my shoulder, making a face. During college she grew accustomed to sleeping in, waking only when her boyfriend came to the room with a cardboard container of sweet and light coffee and a Danish from the Chock full o'Nuts across the street. He always brought the newspapers, too, and he still does; he was such a completely satisfactory boyfriend that he was promoted to husband, although it took a lot of convincing to persuade him to accept the position. I read the paper and do the *New York Times* crossword puzzle. Then I power walk for an hour, almost exactly four miles, either in Riverside Park or on a hilly loop at the house in the country.

And when I get home I call Janet. Not every morning, but most. Sometimes we have lots to discuss, about what we're reading, about what's in the papers, about our families, about our other friends. Sometimes we don't because we've sent each other emails all afternoon the day before, or it's a slow news day, or one or both of us are out of sorts. Only once, in all these years, has my husband said, "What do you and Janet have to talk about? You just talked to her yesterday." It actually was kind of great to hear him say that, because it was such a word-perfect blast from the past. I could hear my father saying the same thing as I lay on the kitchen floor, my feet propped against the wall, curling the long cord of the wall phone around my finger with its ragged bitten nail. This was when talking on the phone was different than it is for my children, when a cellphone was the kind of thing you saw in a sci-fi film, when a cordless phone was a phone that wouldn't work, when there were only one or two phones in the entire house and God forbid you used one to make a long-distance call, even to one of your friends at the Jersey shore, because if it was person to person instead of station to station it would cost real money and show up on the bill and your parents would say "Long distance?!" as though you'd piled money on the patio and set it afire.

"What do you and Donna have to talk about?" my father would say. "You just saw her at school." Sometimes he'd just hang the phone up, and I'd stalk off and slam the bedroom door. "Don't slam that door," my father would shout.

Donna was my best friend, what my daughter calls her bestie, what is now referred to as a BFF, or Best Friend Forever. Who knows what we talked about? The Beatles, her older sisters, Robert Ferreri, Mother Marie Therese, the matinee upcoming at the Waverly Theatre, what we wanted for Christmas. When we moved away, it was leaving Donna that was the worst part. And that's just how I feel about Janet today. Neither one of us likes it much when the other goes on vacation. For most women my age, friends are an essential part of our daily lives— the phone calls, the emails, the coffee, the lunch, the glass of wine. Today we have the time. Once I threw cereal bowls on the table and stuffed gym clothes into backpacks in the morning, rushing out the door, always late, telling myself I owed a phone call here, a card there, and I would get around to it in a few days, which became a few weeks, and even sometimes months. But I don't do that anymore.

When I was young I used to make fun of older couples, with the two guys in the front seat of the car and the two women in the back, used to wrinkle my nose at parties where the men were in the living room with beers and the women in the kitchen filling platters with cold cuts. But now I totally get it. I love hanging out with other women. It's just that feeling that there's someone not obliged by bonds of blood or marriage to support, advise, and love you. My kids learned long ago to like a feather bed atop the mattress, and that's how I think of friendship. Even if your life is comfortable, it's great to have some extra cushioning.

The women I know who are happiest today are the ones who have close female friends. Maybe that's true of men, too, but essentially it's different. I used to have a line in a speech about my editor's advice to write columns about what I was talking about with my friends on the telephone. "If my husband had to write a column based on his phone calls with friends . . ." I would begin, but I never got to finish the sentence because every woman in the audience would start laughing. They all knew that male phone conversations were designed to make plans, while their own were intended to deconstruct the world.

One study of college students showed that both men and women valued friendship, but they were deeply divergent when asked what friendship entailed. Guys thought it meant doing things together, women that it meant emotional sharing and talking. Another study showed that while stress produced the old familiar fight-or-flight response in men—or, as we women often think of it, lash out or shut down—it produces what the researchers termed a tend-or-befriend effect in women. When things go wrong, they reach for either the kids or the girlfriends. Or both.

In other words, friends are what we women have in addition to, or in lieu of, therapists. And when we reach a certain age, they may be who is left. An analysis of census results shows that more than half of all American women are living without a spouse, because of either choice or circumstances. While marriage was once the norm and unmarried somewhere between sad and tragic, staying single is now a considered decision for many women, particularly those who are divorced and feel liberated by being on their own. My single sister has the best take on this one; once, when asked why she was still unmarried years after the end of a brief marriage, she responded, thinking about her ability to do what she likes when she likes, "It would take a helluva man to replace no man at all." Or maybe I should quote the contentedly divorced woman who told a reporter for *The*

New York Times, "One night I slept on the other side of the bed, and I thought, I like this side."

My daughter and her friends are better at this friendship stuff in a lot of ways than we were. They have the same mean-girl gene that we had, at the same time—Maria once told me she was worried about having a daughter someday herself because of having to get her through seventh and eighth grade relatively unscathed. But they are more honest than I remember being, willing to confront one another about disloyalty or bad behavior. Perhaps it's a function of their upbringing during a time when talk show guests regularly argued about their family relationships and marriages, when it's become gospel that silence is not golden but toxic. When I once mentioned that among my youthful girlfriends the idea of having an intervention about a slight would have been unthinkable, Maria was incredulous. "How did you work stuff out?" she asked. "We didn't," I replied.

They are savvy enough to understand that there are friendships worth fighting for. And sometimes, of course, there are those that are not. Over the course of our lives friends fall away, sometimes because they were never really more than friendly acquaintances, sometimes because of differences in circumstance. There were friends we lost when we had children and they did not, and friends we lost and then found again when they had children of their own. There are those divorces in which one friend was chosen over another, and those remarriages in which the chosen friend drifts away because the new spouse is hostile or threatened.

And in the end we wind up with the friends who really stick. Being female, we pride ourselves on doing for them, on listening to them complain or cry, on showing up with a cake or a casserole and taking charge when disaster strikes. But the measure of our real friends, our closest friends, is that we let them do the same for us. We've been taking charge for decades; to let go, to take help instead of charge, is the break point of friendship. And it comes to us, finally, when we are older and wiser, when we've got bigger things to think about than where to buy a coffee table or whether the new guy at work will be collegial. One of the most important parts of tending our friendships is working our way, over time, into the kind of friendships that can support cataclysm, friendships that are able to move from the office or the playground to hospital rooms and funerals. Some of my married friends are widows now, and some are single, and some have lost parents and had kids who were lost to them for a while. And even those of us who so far have been relatively unscathed know how important the bonds of love are, how they make a net so we don't hit the ground when we fall from the wire. We've all prevailed on the individuality front, know without thinking that we are distinct, specific, perhaps even at this time in our lives a little on the eccentric side. So we're free to embrace community, that sense of being part of something bigger and more powerful than ourselves. Or perhaps it's that we stand between two enormous forces. On the one side are the difficult and demanding events to come, the losses, the illnesses, the deaths. You can see them out on the horizon like a great wave, its whitecaps approaching. But on the other hand is a levee that protects us, that of the women we can call anytime, day or night, to say, "I'm drowning here."

And so the morning goes like this: at some point I say to Janet, "I'll talk to you tomorrow." It's not that there's anything really to discuss. Or maybe there will be. Maybe over those twenty-four hours one of us will have bad news, or just a bad day, or something great will have happened and we can crow over it together. Maybe the scaffolding of professional confidence will sag, or one of our other friends will be hurting, or hurt us. Or maybe we will just have one of those desultory conversations friends have: What are you doing? Not much. How's your cold? Better. What's on for tonight? Nothing.

What will we talk about? What did we talk about? Who knows? Who cares? It's the presence at the other end of the line that matters: reliable, loving, listening, caring, continuing. What would I do without her?

PART II

The Wisdom of Why

I should have liked, I do confess, to have had the lightest license of a child and yet been man enough to know its value.

—CHARLES DICKENS,
A Christmas Carol

When we were in college one ubiquitous bumper sticker read, QUESTION AUTHORITY. It was a good piece of advice, but at the time we interpreted it too narrowly: don't trust the power structure, the politicians, the parents.

Today we have a fuller, more satisfying sense of the meaning of those words. We're unlearning so many lessons, about how we should live, be, work, feel. We hold our fingers up to the prevailing winds of custom and behavior and think, nope, that's an ill wind. It's not that we question authority, it's that we question who gets to be an authority in the first place. The notion of what it means to be a woman, a mother, even a human being, has changed so much during our lifetimes. For every incarnation there was a set of shalt nots, and as each became obsolete, we became more skeptical about the commandments. Who says? By what authority? Why this way and not that one?

For me, one of the greatest glories of growing older is the willingness to ask why and, getting no good answer, deciding to follow my own inclinations and desires. Asking why is the way to wisdom. Why are we supposed to want possessions we don't need and work that seems besides the point and tight shoes and a fake tan? Why are we supposed to think new is better than old, youth and vigor better than long life and experience? Why are we supposed to turn our backs on those who have preceded us and to snipe at those who come after?

It's a sure bet that when we were small children we asked "Why?" constantly. Why is the sky blue? Why does the stove burn? Why can't we eat grass? Then, of course, it was a constant voyage of discovery, parsing the known universe by inches. Asking the question now is more a matter of testing the limits of what sometimes seems a narrow world, a world of unrealistic expectations, of conventional wisdom. One of the useful things about age is realizing that conventional wisdom is often simply inertia with a candy coating of conformity.

It's funny how this works. When we're little we want to do what we want to do when we want to do it. Slowly but surely we learn to set our body clocks to some standard time. Then a moment arrives when we learn to say "Why?" again, and to balk if the answer is unsatisfactory. Maybe it's because we know there's no heft behind the consequences; at this point if someone says to me, "You can't do that," I'm perfectly capable of smiling, shrugging, and going full speed ahead. The hard-and-fast rules don't seem so hard and fast. That's how we get a handle on what we want to keep and what we can afford to jettison. There's a fearlessness to our lives now that comes from knowing that the authorities we can accept and trust are close to home: the women who went before us, the friends who confide and support, the voice inside that says, Ah, go ahead. What have you got to lose?

Generations

I've learned the most about myself, these last few years, by looking back, not at my own life but at my place in the succession of women who came before me. For so long I sold them short. My mother, for instance. My mother was a housewife, a rather reserved person with a sweet nature and a powerful ability to control her children through the simple exigency of spontaneous and utterly sincere tears. That was how I pigeonholed her for many years, her and many others like her.

But the truth was that once upon a time my mother had been someone else. I know this because there are photographs of her, in Lana Turner shorts, wasp-waisted against a fence post on her honeymoon. There was the occasional story about a before-Bob boyfriend, terrifying in the implication that we might have never been born, or been born only half ourselves, passing the other half in Wanamaker's at Christmastime.

But mainly I know this because of the drafting table in the basement. I wish I had it now, glossy wood, tilt top, talismanic. Apparently for a short time after high school my mother worked as a draftsman—that's what she said, draftsman, not draftswoman—at General Electric. My father says she was the only woman there, that they erected something they called a maiden veil at the front of her drafting table, a modesty panel designed to safeguard her dignity because in those days all working women wore skirts. I wish I had asked her about it, if the guys gave her a hard time, if she rued trading the job in for marriage and multiple pregnancies. But I never did.

I thought of myself as a woman who had burst free of the circle of Avon Lady, Tupperware Party, and Fuller Brush Man that my mother inhabited, not someone who was the daughter of a woman who was the first or only of her profession. That version of my mother seemed less real to me than Jo March in *Little Women*. The mother I knew spent years in maternity smocks and seemed to iron incessantly. I don't own an iron, never have, and that's no accident. The combination of hot metal and a damp dress shirt seemed to me to be a sentence to a life of nothing much. I couldn't imagine what my mother did all day, even when there was a new baby in the house to care for and stew on the table for dinner and clean uniform blouses in my closet. That's the point of being a kid, the kind of magical thinking that suggests that the details of your existence just sort of happen. But sometimes I think that my entire generation of women adopted, for a time, that childlike point of view, that the women who raised us did things that were tedious and beneath notice.

You had only to listen to us to know that this was true, listen to our implied belief in our own singularity. We invented natural childbirth. Also toilet training and time-outs and open communication and story time. We invented balancing work and family, and spousal divisions of labor, and sexual harassment and equal pay for equal work. Or at least we behaved as though we had. Occasionally someone would call us on all this. Once, when I wrote a column about juggling writing and childrearing, a mother of six who had taught high school Spanish for fifty years wrote me a mildly peremptory letter suggesting that discussions by baby boomer women might occasionally reflect that they were not the first humans ever to have both a job and children. A Southern lady in her nineties sent me six pages of scented flowered stationery detailing all the ways in which we liked to imply that children before our own had been raised by wolves.

Ah, the interplay of the generations, part internecine warfare, part uneasy coexistence. How different it seems viewed from one end or the other. We have all been part of the great unbroken generational chain of younger people who believe they could do much better than those who came before them. And then one day we wake to discover that we are the older women we once discounted, and our perspective shifts. Younger people came along to criticize their elders, and their elders happened to be us.

From natural childbirth to discipline without corporal punishment, from sex education to gender equity, those of us of a certain age spent decades suggesting, even openly opining, that our mothers were a bit behind the curve. We sat in the living room and talked about how breast was best, how Lamaze breathing worked, how reading to babies would pay off. It is a tribute to the patience and the discretion of our aunts, grandmothers, neighbors, and mothers that, in the main, they did not reply, "Oh, girls, get over yourselves."

Perhaps because of the changes in the lives of women during our formative years, we grew up thinking of ourselves as distinct, even special. The good news is that we outgrew this, one of the clearest benefits of getting older. It's true that my mother fed her babies food from jars while I made the food for my own. It's also true that she didn't have a sitter five days a week, that she couldn't call for takeout when all five of us were clamoring for dinner, takeout being one of the unexpected linchpins of female freedom in our time. The closest thing my mother had to a windup baby bouncer was her arm and hip.

What of my aunt Kay, who always seemed cool and composed and beautifully put together although she had eight children, or even my grandmother, whom I remember as slightly indolent and self-absorbed, a Manhattan at her dimpled elbow as she sat in the living room in a floral print dress and talked about Clover Day sales at Strawbridge and Clothier? One of her sons was taken prisoner during World War II. One of her daughters died as a toddler, on the same day, in the same hospital, as she was giving birth to yet another son, my father. She shopped. She endured. I was stopped cold by this description of the effects of World War II from the memoirs of the Duchess of Devonshire, a woman with blue bloodlines and a manor house that makes Buckingham Palace look like government offices: "Two of my brothers-in-law; my only brother; Andrew's only brother; my four best friends—all killed within a month of each other." How does a woman recover from that? I wonder now how we dared to criticize and condescend to a generation of women who soldiered on through the Depression, a world war, and a world without much in the way of family planning or job opportunities.

Of course we now accept that they were heroines, the ones who mothered so many. And so were the ones who worked when married women weren't expected to work at all, and unmarried women who took jobs as secretaries and nurses and teachers, paid less and yet happy to be paid at all. When the doors busted open, the doors to medical and law schools, many smart women my age were contemptuous of what had been traditional female jobs. Medicine meant being a doctor. Education meant being a university professor. We wanted to have a secretary, not be one. Eventually we learned that that was short-sighted. The most pivotal figure in a birthing room is the labor-and-delivery nurse. Our children spent more time with their teachers on any given day than they did with us.

We were climbing on the shoulders of the women who had gone before us, but it was not just we who were elevated, but the entire enterprise. More women on the staffs and mastheads of the country's largest publications, for instance, changed those publications for the better. In the beginning most female reporters were employed on the social pages, which featured recipes and dress patterns and fashion coverage and wedding announcements. One or two would slip through the net and cover Washington or City Hall, Paris or London. And eventually covering Washington led to covering the White House—the president, not the First Lady. The lives of women changed, and so did the women's pages, and so did the women's assignments, and the final product. Newspapers became more reflective of the world around them, and therefore better.

When we looked at the women who had preceded us, in law or medicine or business or education or most other fields, we realized that they had been engaged in an essential kabuki dance of gender and status. There was scorn attached to this, once it was safe to be female, employed, and ambitious: one of our older colleagues was "passing," another had prospered by being "one of the boys." In my office the woman who seemed to exemplify this other world, this world before us, was a woman named Charlotte Curtis, who had edited the women's pages and then the opinion pages of *The New York Times*. Some of the young female reporters confused how she looked with who she was; she dressed like one of the women she had skewered in her sharp society coverage, in skirt suits, heels, heavy gold jewelry, her hair perfectly arranged, a hat of hair. It was understood that she was not one of us. She ran with the men of management, she would not rock the boat of careful gender arrangements, she had become the first woman on the *Times* masthead by going along to get along.

Which made it all the more surprising to me when she asked me to lunch at Sardi's restaurant, when I had been appointed the first woman deputy metropolitan editor. She asked me politely about myself and at some point in the meal uttered a sentence that I will always remember: "You should never forget that you will only have as much power as they are willing to give you." She recognized that I was full of myself, full of the gains and advances of my youth, full of the notion that women had progressed past the point of needing to be one of the boys. She wanted me to understand that men still set the agenda, that progress was relative, that the certainty of youth is often rooted in oversimplification. Surely my misunderstanding of Charlotte Curtis should have taught me something: Robin Morgan, in her memoir, *Saturday's Child,* recounted the story behind the scenes of the feminist protest at the Miss America pageant in 1968 and of how Charlotte, of all people, had secretly provided the money to bail out those who had been busted for disrupting the live telecast. "She was what they used to call 'a real lady,'" wrote Robin, revealing the secret. "But she was a real feminist, too."

The writer Jane O'Reilly published a wonderful piece in *Ms.* magazine when I was in college titled "The Housewife's Moment of Truth," in which she detailed the indignities of being female that made a *click!* go off in our heads. I can barely count my own clicks over the years, although I'm particularly attached to the moment when I tried to persuade the registrar of the hospital that my surname was different from that of my husband and therefore different from that of our newborn child, and she tried to persuade me that I might as well just save everyone a lot of trouble and adopt my husband's last name when I signed the birth certificate forms. "This is where most of you girls fold," she'd said without malice as blind rage bloomed in my chest. Or maybe that was my milk coming in, combined with the blind rage.

But there's another moment of truth I've learned to recognize, and it's the moment when we realize that other people, often other women, often women of another generation, are not what we so conveniently expect them to be. It's that moment when we realize that we—we!—were prejudiced, that we lapsed into stereotype based on sex. It's what I felt when I learned about Charlotte Curtis paying the bail money. It's what I felt when I talked with an eighty-year-old about her abortion, or discussed strategy with a woman who was once a union organizer. "I learned to play them like a violin," she said of her male peers.

How did I forget for so many years about my mother's drafting table? Where did it go? My father says my mother kept it because after she was done having children (was she ever done having children?) she intended to do freelance work from home. That never happened. She didn't live long enough. If she had, maybe she would have been a draftsman again. Or, this time, a draftswoman. Or something else entirely.

Some of the women of my mother's generation got married and had children and then eventually did go back to work. Some of them chose not to have families at all despite the standards of their time, brave enough to go up against the assumption that they would inevitably be incomplete, unhappy. Some of them were beaten down by societal expectations and bored to tears in the houses their husbands bought and paid for, and who can blame them? Others liked that life just fine, and they've gotten quite tired of hearing that they wasted their time.

It must tickle them to watch those of us who had the advantages they were denied suddenly finding the tables turned. Now, finally, we understand the challenges they faced; now, finally, we face some of the same disdain from younger women that they faced from us. At one college a smart young woman stood up and told me pugnaciously that she would be marrying early, having kids quickly, staying home to care for them in the way that only their mother could, entering the workplace afterward. She and her friends had heard enough about epidemic infertility, nanny horror stories, the difficulties of finding a partner later in life. They would not make the same mistakes we made, she said, to some applause.

Karma is a boomerang, and a bitch.

Some of my friends and colleagues are enraged by young women like this, who pick away at the lives that were so hard-won, who blithely say they know better. Maybe because I was once some facsimile of that selfsame self-satisfied girl, pontificating about refusing to do stereotypically female stories, inveighing against the barbarity of the obstetrical episiotomy even before I'd gotten pregnant (and then, in late-stage labor, begging for one), I have more patience. The young women who follow us have a point. I know many of my peers who feel they waited too long to have children, even know some who think they were too choosy about who and when and whether to marry. When I was helping to run the metro desk and female reporters would confide that they were pregnant and then rattle off what sounded like a travel itinerary of due date, maternity leave, and return to work, I would caution them to wait and see whether they wanted to come right back or take more time. We hadn't realized yet that motherhood is a various thing.

But that student detailing her plans for the future, plans based on the imagined shortcomings of the lives lived by women like me, had yet to learn how various life can be. She, too, was making the mistake of bringing a cookie-cutter approach to the future, as other generations had done before her. It was just a different cookie. It didn't seem useful to tell her that younger moms might have less patience and experience, that sometimes taking care of children full time felt like a cross between a carnival ride and penal servitude, that she would be surprised at how many potential employers would consider the resulting gap on her résumé to be a deal breaker. Often it feels as though generations shout at one another across a canyon with roaring water at the bottom, drowning out the words. Somehow, eventually, we find our way. When we are kids we craft that way in opposition to our elders. And then when we are older we look back at the opposition and think how foolish some of it was.

Somehow I think the canyon dividing the generations is deeper for women. And it's not simply the young passing judgment on those of us who have gone before. We return the favor. Creeping codgerism is an inevitable effect of getting older, a variation of memory loss, the rich tradition of adults insisting that the younger generation has slalomed through an easy life while their generation pushed the rock of responsibility uphill. When I complain that my daughter's skirt looks more like a belt, or that my sons keep vampire hours, those are the churlish carpings of a woman years removed from the days when her own hems were sky-high and her idea of a good time was sleeping until noon.

Yet if there has ever been an American generation that ought to know better than to trash the young, to question their clothes and their music and their work habits and their hair, it is we baby boomers. We single-handedly turned aging from a life cycle into a political and moral failing. When, almost half a century ago, the children of the United States embraced pacifism, civil rights, the liberation of women, and a sexual revolution, they did it largely by demonizing their parents' generation as avatars of war, prejudice, and prudery. With what glee those parents, now in their eighties, could greet the sight of so many of us muting or abandoning our counterculture principles! Abbie Hoffman, nearing his fiftieth birthday, turned the slogan "Don't trust anyone over thirty" on its head and criticized a new generation of college students for their lack of activism, saying that he'd learned not to trust anyone *under* thirty. Roger Daltrey, the lead singer of the band the Who, at least had the good sense not to sing the famous line "Hope I die before I get old" as, pushing seventy, he performed during halftime at the Super Bowl. We have become the older generation we once inveighed against. And we can, like generations before us, approach that in one of two ways. We can gracefully accept and embrace changing mores. Or we can dig in our heels and pretend that we know best. We can be role models, or old coots.

Before we talk about how much easier the next generation has it, we might consider this: In 1974 I graduated from a prestigious liberal arts college. I'd paid my own way the last two years with jobs as a dormitory resident assistant and a newspaper summer intern. I rented a small, charming, cheap one-bedroom apartment in lower Manhattan and started work as a reporter the Monday after commencement. Only a fool would think that kind of experience is possible today. To earn the money to pay for a year at a fine liberal arts college, a student would have to have a summer job robbing banks. There are no cheap one-bedroom apartments in lower Manhattan. In fact, the monthly rent today on my former apartment is probably about the same as my total annual tuition in 1974. My youth seems not difficult but idyllic compared to what many younger people face. When I told my children that I had taken the SAT just once, without resorting to a prep class, and that I had done no community service to flesh out my college application, they were gobsmacked.

Given the fact that the American dream is that children outstrip their parents—ditch digger to cop to judge in three generations of an Irish immigrant family—and that that dream now seems out of reach, my children's generation are remarkably good-humored. Given the pressures we've put upon them, they're also savvy, and rightly skeptical about some of the choices we've made. If they've seen their elders laid off from a company to which they'd given the best years of their lives, young people may have concluded that loyalty to the corporation is a historical artifact. If they've watched marriages buckle and work tasks displace family time, they may vow to find jobs that accommodate them when they have their own kids. If they've been listening to the drumbeat of burnout, downsizing, and stress, the tom-tom of modern existence, maybe they've decided that they intend to try to have a life life as well as a work life. I, for one, can't argue. My father traveled constantly on business. Is it coincidence that I've somehow finagled a job that allows me to work at home?

It's odd how we approach all those things we want for the next generation, the things we say we value most. We want them to have children of their own, but much of our discussion about childrearing makes it sound difficult and terrifying. We want them to have work they find satisfying, but we complain often about our own jobs. Americans of a certain age are disgruntled about how they are treated by younger people, and to ensure that those younger people understand that growing older carries clear benefits, perspective, experience, freedom, self-awareness, they talk about how horrible it is.

This is one of the surefire ways to tell if you're truly getting older: if you complain constantly both about aging and about how little aging is valued and respected. We all do it, and we all rue it, too. There are other markers of age, of course: lunch conversation about ailments, prescription meds, and surgery, the watching of the Weather Channel and the reading of obituaries. The obvious antidotes: a shaggy haircut, a sharp jacket, and downloaded music.

My own mother used to totally rock out to my brother Bob's Led Zeppelin albums, and the very fact that I offer that example today illustrates another problem of aging: the terror that you're turning into what you once considered the lamest aspects of your parents. When was the first time I did this? I can't remember the exact occasion, only the physical sensation of uncomfortable recognition, even horror. My words hung in the air, echoing through a filmy curtain of déjà vu: "Because I said so." I also said, "Wait until your father gets home." I said, "Your face will freeze like that." Now I'm hoping that lightning will strike me if I ever utter the phrase "When you're my age."

Some lines from my parents' past I can't use; they are past their sell-by date. Please get your hair out of your eyes, my mother would say, you look like Veronica Lake. That's another hallmark of the divide between the generations, the evocation of cultural landmarks that mean nothing. My daughter looks up from the crossword puzzle and says, "Television show named *My Little* what?" *Margie,* I reply. Vietnamese festival and American military incursion? Tet. Ronald Reagan's attorney general? Meese. The gap between us yawns. One day, doing laundry, it occurred to me that the continuum in which I found myself included the demise of women's underwear. I had stacks of my own bikini pants on top of the dryer, and I was comparing them in my mind to my mother's remembered granny panties and my daughter's own barely-there lace thongs. If you laid that lingerie in a line, it not only gave you a road map of the differences in sexual mores and openness through the years, it also suggested that the next generation of young women, my granddaughters, would wind up going commando. "Ew," Maria said when I shared my thoughts with her. I imagined her begging her own daughters to wear underpants, throwing up her hands and saying "Your grandmother said it would come to this" while her girls rolled their eyes dismissively: Oh, well, Nana. She's ancient. What does she know?

The similarities echo down the years as each group learns from and then dismisses its elders, as each group passes judgment on the one that comes after. We insist on talking about why young people will never amount to anything, and they insist on talking about all we've done wrong in our lives and how they will do things better. I'm part of the generation that said it wanted to change the world, and it did. We insisted we wanted more than our mothers had, and we got it. We let the forty-hour work week morph into the sixty-hour work week and even the eighty-hour work week, and in between those hours at the desk we had those hours in the kitchen and the car, overseeing homework, making the rounds of athletic fields. For those of us who feared as girls that our lives would be empty and boring, the crazed timpani of our existences at least meant that we were not in some domestic dead end. But I'm not sure, if we are being honest, that we would consider our alternative ideal. I'm developing a certain comfort level with the criticisms of those young women who will make a different sort of life for themselves. If their experience of their exhausted, insomniac, dispirited elders makes them decide they'd prefer not to go straight from the classroom to the cubicle to the coffin, it doesn't necessarily mean they're ungrateful. Maybe it means they're sane.

Or maybe it just means that they're different, and that we can learn from them. Change, as we all know, is the great constant. There's a quote I like from Mark Twain: "They didn't know it was impossible, so they did it!" Remember when we were those people? We were certain that we'd discovered freedom, possibility, new ways of living, loving, raising families. And we were right. Our parents were, too, and the same is true for the generation to come, and so on and so forth.

Near Miss

One evening I sat at her kitchen table with a friend who had been widowed the year before, talking about this and that and how she was getting by, when suddenly she said, "I figure, here's the good news: at least we never got divorced."

I went home that night thinking about what she'd meant by that, whether the marriage had been rocky in its last years, if there'd always been internal upheaval that none of us had seen. But what she meant, of course, was simply that we all have a list of bad things that can happen, dark roads we can wander down, and she'd realized that there was at least one of those that she had avoided forevermore.

We build our lives bit by bit of small bricks, until by the end there's a long stretch of masonry. But one of the amazing, and frightening, things about growing older, about seeing yourself surrounded by the Great Wall of Life, is that you become aware of how random the construction is, how many times it could have gone a different way, the mistakes that you averted, not because you were wise, perhaps, but because you were lucky. You didn't get pregnant when you didn't want to be, and you did when you did, and at the time you think that's just how it is. And then years after, when you consider all the ways in which things went differently for people like you, you wonder.

What if? You can get a whole table of girlfriends going with that one question. What if? If I'd gone to a different college I would never have met my husband, never had this life or these children. If I hadn't been a babysitter for the two couples I chose from the college file box, I wouldn't have gotten that first newspaper job in New York. And that first job led to the next, and the next, and so much that came after. The whole thing holds together; take one brick out and you can see it come tumbling down around your ears.

We often think of turning points as monumental events, but in retrospect they are so often minor moments: a lunch here, a drink there, a chance meeting, a fluke. When we were first married, my husband persuaded me that I could learn to be happy in the suburbs, which reminds me yet again of how clouded your judgment can be when you're young and in love and have been preapproved for a mortgage by the bank. We made an offer on a sweet little house, but the roof, it turned out, was shot, and we walked away. My whole life might have been different if the roof on that house had been sound. I know now that I'm just not a suburban person.

All the stories and songs, they talk about the lost opportunities. "The Ben I'll never be, who remembers him?" asks a character ruefully in the musical *Follies*. And we do have to make our peace with diminished expectations, bit by bit, the road not taken, the role not filled.

But sometimes I think that the emphasis on those moments that have passed us by obscures our gratitude for those pitfalls we skirted. Life is full of close calls, jobs that seemed like a good idea at the time but in retrospect would have been a bust, relationships that were so, so seductive but that today seem like moments of sheer madness. Being smart about life, and about ourselves, means that we know that it wasn't that we were savvy, or strategic; sometimes we just lucked out. Or not.

It's all so random. Some of my good luck, for instance, was that there were lots of bad things I wasn't good at. I took up smoking during a sabbatical from school during which I was working as a newspaper clerk and tormented by doubts about who I was and where I was going. Sometime in the spring the city editor, whose phone I answered and mail I opened, decided I could start doing some stories, and to mark the moment I bought some cigarettes and a leather messenger bag large enough to hold a dozen reporter's notebooks. I smoked the way I swung a bat, as though I was doing a bad imitation of something I'd seen on film: Dunhills, because everyone would take me seriously if I smoked cigarettes that were strong, had no filters, and were imported from England in a burgundy-and-gold box. This was when smoking was not only permitted in newsrooms, it was almost encouraged. In fact, even if I had not smoked, I would have been smoking, given the gray fug that hung over the room. The secondhand smoke probably did more to my lungs than my own passing habit, since I'm pretty sure I never learned to inhale properly.

My history with drugs was even more short-lived and strange, although I was a teenager and then a young single New Yorker just at the moment when so-called soft drugs were in fullest, most conspicuous, most jubilant flower. For years I put the fact that I never dropped acid or snorted coke down to a night, my third time smoking pot, when I apparently got a joint with something stronger in it, became almost terminally paranoid in a bar, went home, pulled the covers over my head, and slept for the better part of a day. I think of it every time George Bailey gets freaked out by Clarence the angel in *It's a Wonderful Life* and brays, "Ernie, straighten me out here, I've got some bad liquor or something." Now it seems like a lucky break, but in the moment I was tormented by the notion that I couldn't even be cool enough to get high.

Over time it developed that my real issue is not that I'm not cool, although that is true. It's that I am what might kindly be called a control freak. This makes me not singular, but typical. The illusion of control is the besetting addiction, and delusion, of the modern age. We now have so much information, so many safeguards, so much statistical data about everything from car crashes to investment formulas that we've convinced ourselves that we can control our environment. Modern life tells us that this is so. Rooms that are always cool even in a desert setting that is mostly over 100 degrees, New York to Beijing in half a day, three-dimensional scans of the heart, online dating, in utero photography: What in the world is not within our grasp? So much information, and information is power, the power to believe that if we follow certain prescriptions, certain events will follow. In other words, life as mathematical equation: If Ivy League, then success. If high fiber, then low cholesterol. If parental involvement, then happy children.

And then the randomness of events intercedes, and the illusion of control crumbles. A pleasant flight attendant, watching me wedge myself against the back of the seat in front of me during a bout of turbulence, once said that she thought I was the kind of person who would be fine with flying if I could just pilot the plane myself. (Never going to happen.) That's what we learn as we grow older: That we are not always piloting the plane. That unexpected things occur. That control is a nice concept, little more.

So we control, in the parlance of the prayer, the things we can, which usually means inanimate objects, and ourselves. I'm that woman who had the hysterectomy with local anesthesia. General anesthesia is for some of us with control issues what being locked in a basement closet is for claustrophobics. So I found a doctor who was not only uncommonly gifted and highly recommended but also willing to operate with only a local epidural anesthetic to render me numb from the waist down. Because she had met with me on several occasions, she had one proviso: "You can't talk to me while I'm operating." Because you know I wanted to.

I acquired a guided-imagery tape narrated by a woman named Belleruth Naparstek, whose name I will never forget because you never forget the person talking inside your head as you're looking up at the big lights in the operating room. She gave me the impression that I could control what was going on. She told me to imagine my body helping to heal itself, to imagine all the people I loved standing around the surgical table. She told me I might become emotional, even weepy, and I thought, Oh, hooey! as I imagined my mother and my kids—I'm sorry, but I just didn't think my husband and father could handle it—circling the table on my side of the surgical drape. That was something else: the surgeon said I couldn't watch her. Because you know I wanted to.

"Anything above the waist, you're going to have to have a general," she said kindly afterward, perhaps recognizing me as a special kind of superannuated control freak.

I wonder—does every control freak have something they clearly cannot control? For me that something was booze. I love booze. Or at least I think I do. I've now spent more of my adult life without it than I did with it, so it's difficult to tell. Maybe it's like that old boyfriend you remember so fondly; if you met him again, you might still think he is handsome, witty, so much fun. Or you might wonder: What was I thinking? Scotch tastes like turpentine. Wine is nothing but an invitation to stomach acid.

Do all of us, by the time we're grown-ups, have something that was our signal lucky break? Sometimes it's marrying someone, sometimes divorcing them. Sometimes it's finding a lump when it's small, or getting the meds that turned a ravening monster of depression into a medium-size dog on a short leash. Sometimes it's getting lost on a back road and passing a house with a FOR SALE sign.

For me it was giving up booze, and giving it up early. None of my three adult children has the faintest memory of Mommy pounding down a bottle of wine or a six-pack, which of course is why I stopped in the first place when my youngest was a baby. I think parents are often confusing for kids—I discovered the other day that my eldest can recite from memory the excellent Philip Larkin poem that begins "They fuck you up, your mum and dad," despite the fact that he allegedly thinks we are good parents—and I therefore think it's much too hard for any child to have several mothers over the course of a single evening. "My mother was a drunk" is one of the harshest, saddest sentences in any language.

I'm doubly aware of this now, at my age, so many years past that last drink—a Heineken beer—because I've begun to realize how bad habits seem worse when the habitué is of a certain age. We harden as we grow older; our behaviors are less watercolor, more etching: The control freak becomes an obsessive. That charming guy who can't help himself, who hits on virtually any woman with a pulse, is a stud at thirty-five and nothing but a terrible lech thirty years later. The woman who has always been an inveterate storyteller begins to seem, when she's aged, nothing more than a garrulous pain. And the lively, charismatic, sociable thirty-year-old who regaled the entire bar with terrific stories over the course of a long night becomes, as time goes by, nothing more than an object of pity. His friends lower their voices, lean in hard: "He drinks." What was once a description is now an indictment.

The truth is that if I'd gone to AA meetings, I wouldn't have had very much to say. I never drove into anything, never missed work, never fell into a restaurant table or threw up at a dinner party. But one day in the dentist's office I found myself taking a quiz in a woman's magazine about whether you had a drinking problem. And with a blinding flash of *duh!* I understood that if you were even bothering to take the test, you already knew the answer. I was one of those women who were exquisitely sensitive to how others saw them, who spent all their time looking over their shoulder at themselves. That's a form of contortionism that comes at a cost. I suppose I loosened up when I drank and stopped, like the White Rock girl, looking at me looking at me looking at me.

With age I truly stopped doing that, stopped worrying so much in every crowded room about whether I was wearing the wrong dress, saying the wrong thing, making the wrong impression. So perhaps I would have slowly become one of those creatures, miraculous to me, who can nurse one glass of white wine for an evening. But maybe not. Moderation and I have always had an uneasy relationship. And perhaps that's truer now than ever. It may be that all people become more of whatever they mostly are as they grow older, the good as well as the bad: more outspoken, less inhibited, funnier, more gregarious. Sometimes it seems as though age strips away the furbelows, the accessories, and leaves just the essential person, the same way that as you get older you learn to dispense with ruffles and fancy buttons and just wear a black sheath dress. I had an aunt who, among other things, was known for a tongue so sharp that it sometimes qualified as a lethal weapon. As she developed dementia and her world shrank to a pinhole view, like that last frame in a Looney Tunes cartoon, she recognized no one but her husband and she lost most of her personality except for the occasional whipsaw of sharp words.

I think of giving up drinking as a little like passing an intersection where someone has blown through the red light, smashing up his own life and that of whoever was in that crumpled can of a subcompact, realizing as I survey the carnage that if I'd left the house a minute earlier it could have been me: got lucky, beat the reaper, just in time. But, looking around at the landscape of my friendship circles, I don't think that's specific to alcohol abstinence. So many of us know where the fault lines lay, the things we managed to do, or change, or avoid, almost without knowing what we were doing, or why. All the things that, looking back, meant the difference between one life and another. It's why a certain kind of movie has always been so popular, the one that includes a chance encounter on a train or the near miss in the revolving door. Life is haphazard. We plan, and then we deal when the plans go awry. Control is an illusion; best intentions are the best we can do. I remember imagining that I could chart a course that would take me from one place to another. I thought I had a handle on my future. But the future, it turns out, is not a tote bag.

Many years ago I decided that I didn't want to be any worse than my shortcomings made me if I could possibly help it. At the end of a dim tunnel I could see the possibility of a life in which I would be defined not by who I was but by what went from a bottle into a glass and then into my mouth. Worse still, I imagined the lives of those I loved being defined by it as well. It's not insignificant, the number of people who have said to me over the years, with a particular kind of anguished thrum to their voices, "My mother had a drinking problem." But it's a terrible mistake to think that taking care of one thing is taking care of all things. I'm not sure if it's true, but an AA stalwart once told me that more marriages broke up after sobriety than before, simply because it became obvious that the booze wasn't the problem, the relationship was. One of my friends once said sadly of her mother, who had stopped drinking, "I thought she was mean because she drank. But she's just mean."

Giving up booze didn't change my life in any essential way. I did things that were stupid and things that were thoughtless, even sometimes at parties without the excuse of having had one too many. It turned out that I'm loud even when I'm not drunk, and it turns out that I feel like I'm hungover when I simply haven't gotten enough sleep. There's pretty good alcohol-free champagne for New Year's Eve, although it wouldn't fool anyone who drinks real champagne. For a long time I substituted caffeine for alcohol, although I like to say that no one ever crashed into another car and killed its occupants after having a double espresso with a latte chaser.

Now, in one of those cruel tricks of biology, I drink much less coffee because my aging body has become so sensitive to caffeine that if I have so much as a piece of chocolate cake after noon I will find myself buzzing at midnight. My substitute for alcohol today is what my kids have learned to call fizzy water, which is carbonated water at an absurd markup. At restaurants in Europe they refer to it as *avec gaz,* which always makes me a little uneasy. If I had known when I was young that three-dollar water and five-dollar coffee would become not simply popular but commonplace, I might have gone into a different line of work. But, like most people, I was dumber then. I remember teaching myself, as a young woman, to like the taste of scotch. But now I've forgotten it.

Mirror, Mirror

So many decades looking into the mirror as my eyes look back at me, and I'm still not sure precisely what I'm seeing or how I feel about the result. Especially now. More than anything, it is our faces that tell us the story of the passage of time. We never actually see them the way others do, which may be why we care so deeply what others see when they look at us. The mirror is a poor second to the real thing because it's not transactional, only ourselves facing an inanimate object. Over the years we've learned to edit what we see.

Every face is both a mystery and an identity. We realize this when we try to capture a face in a photograph. It is like taking a picture of the sunset. What you wind up with is a trite arrangement of pink sky and pillowy clouds when what you felt was something else, something greater. Whenever I see a picture of myself I have the same feeling I have when I hear my own voice recorded: My senses have played a trick on me. My ears say I don't sound like that. My eyes say I don't look like that.

But I do. In some way I always have. I suppose it's my good

fortune now to have always had the prominent nose, the square jaw, that seem much more suited to an older woman, or how we think of an older woman. Perhaps part of the reason I've been relatively sanguine about aging is because my face was never my fortune, and it was never really young. And, to be frank, I was never pretty. Cute sometimes, when I was younger. Handsome on occasion, as I aged. But not pretty. "Pretty is what changes" goes the Sondheim song. My face hasn't changed as much as it might have, not because I've aged well but because I've aged into how I always looked.

Not long ago I read a biography of Mary Anne Evans, more commonly known as George Eliot, that suggested she'd written *Middlemarch,* one of the greatest novels in the English language, because she was so unattractive, that had she been more pleasing to look at she would have married, had a brace of children, settled in the English countryside, never become George Eliot at all. Instead she got the message that she would need to use her mind to make up for her face. In other words, a woman can have a Cupid's-bow mouth or an enduring literary reputation, but not both. In the long term most of us will take the reputation, but sadly, in the short term the pretty mouth is what's desired.

This simplistic characterization of George Eliot's life makes a crazy kind of sense for many women. It's the apotheosis of personality in lieu of prettiness that we girls have known about since we cleared the hurdle of fifth grade and our features began to sharpen and harden. Or perhaps I'm hypersensitive because I myself am a person who grew up with the message that I might want to keep on reading those books and honing that mind. As a girl I had the strongly marked face of a grown woman, fourteen cut out to be forty. Which, by the time I was actually forty, was quite a good thing.

This is one of the trade-offs of aging or, if you're what I once called the chocolate-box girls, one of the tragedies. One group grows into their faces and another grows out of them. Well into her eighties, my grandmother used to reprise the days when she was hotly sought after on the Atlantic City boardwalk, a pink-skinned pretty young woman with fair hair waving around her face. As any actress knows, being the ingénue is risky business, short-lived and undependable. A character actress has a much longer shelf life.

When the British actress Harriet Walter curated an exhibit of photographs of older women, she wrote, "Young women and girls are conditioned to aspire to look like other people." One study showed that as many as eight out of ten women are unhappy about their own appearance, while men are either delighted or agnostic about their own; in fact, one study of men showed that some of them overestimate their attractiveness.

Meanwhile, what passes for the baseline for women has become increasingly impossible. More and more obituaries are using photographs of the deceased at a much younger age than the one at which he or she died. And women were twice as likely to do this, which means either they were convinced that the world should see them for the last time in their physical prime, or their family was, or they'd refused to have their picture taken after they'd reached a certain age.

The business of appearance stops being a level playing field some time after college, when suddenly a man's face is less important than his professional stature and bank balance. Who among us has not seen the photos of a short bald man with the face of a basset hound and an arm around a young creature who would have been declared a goddess in some ancient culture? On the other hand, a woman's professional stature continues to be paired with her appearance, so that it is still commonplace to see descriptions of captains of industry that include hair, suit, and shoes in the unlikely event that the captain of industry is female. There will usually be a mention of her children, too, if she is a mother. If she quits, it will be said that she wanted to spend more time with her family. Sometimes this is even true.

In terms of my own appearance it has been instructive to have a daughter around the house. There are two ways to go if you are lucky enough to have one: You can resent the fact that she easily, effortlessly, has what you once had, that no matter how hard you exercise she will look better than you in a bathing suit, that she rubs on face cream despite the fact that it is manufactured with the promise of giving her exactly the sort of skin she already has. Or you can let her appearance release you from something, something challenging but reassuring, too. You can embrace the fact that you are not that person anymore, with all its surface rewards and all its internal battles. I suppose you could make the argument that various professionals could narrow the gap between the young woman and the older one. Lift it, tuck it, laser it, dye it. You've seen those photos, of the mother and daughter whose time line has been narrowed through the blandishments of many professionals. Except that if you look closely it hasn't, not really. A very famous actress, a woman whose restaurant meals and shopping trips are constantly punctuated with fan babblings and requests for autographs, notes that when she wants to move around the city unmolested, she merely walks with her daughters in a phalanx in front of her. "It's better than sunglasses," she says. Even her golden aura disappears in the shadow of youth.

Her girls and my own have something no colorist, no dermatologist, no makeup artist, no surgeon can provide. It's simple: they look as though they've just been taken out of the gift box, just unwrapped from the tissue and the ribbons. In other words, they're young. Of course, that means they're too young to appreciate the unsolicited gifts that that brings. I remember all the impedimenta we rushed toward, openhanded, that we thought would make us grown-up, or at least female: the stockings, the heels, the makeup, all part of this horrible pantomime. It says everything that they are the things we begin to throw off as we grow older. The heels are uncomfortable, the makeup aging. I hate control-top panty hose. They were invented by sadists.

All the plastic surgery in the world cannot conceal the fact that the smooth taut skin of a twenty-year-old is lost to a fifty-year-old, whose body and face show length of service. When I began my annual pilgrimage to the Fountain of Botox—later supplemented with one to the Shrine of Facial Fillers—it wasn't to make me look young again. I'm not that delusional, and no doctor is that skilled. It was to make me look less crabby. The 11 between my brows, the furrows from the corners of my nose to the corners of my mouth: in photographs I could see that they made me look as if I was in a very bad mood. And I wasn't. Now my appearance matches my affect, if not my thirties.

We don't really have any idea of how we ought to look anymore, just how we're told we ought to want to look. Women were once permitted a mourning period for their youthful faces; it was called middle age. Now we don't even have that. Instead we have the science of embalming disguised as grooming. A lot of plastic surgery is like spray tan. It doesn't look like a real tan at all. It looks like a tan in an alternate universe in which everyone is orange. It's a universe in which it seems no one has gray hair, except for me.

When I was young my mother spent a lot of time on my hair. Although I spent hours complaining, wriggling in a dining room chair, sometimes sitting on a phone book or two, deep down I liked it. It was single-minded attention from a person who was frequently pulled in so many directions that she was psychologically drawn and quartered. In the mirror above the sideboard I would see her staring down at my part, like the bright dividing line on the highway. I felt sorry for those girls who went to the hairdresser before the prom, and not simply because half the time they were so appalled at the result, the hair equivalent of those big ugly funeral flower arrangements, that they pulled it all down and raked a brush through the sticky teased mess. My mother did my hair to match my dress. The yellow eyelet with the puffed sleeves called for long waves with the sides lifted into a grosgrain bow, the navy and white empire-waisted dress required something sleeker, a tight bun at the base of my neck capped by a snood dotted with pearls. No hairdresser would ever look out for my hair the way my mother did, and so I listened carefully to her advice for its care, although eventually I gave up on the Alberto VO5.

But I absorbed her warnings about hair coloring. When she talked about hair coloring, my mother made it sound like communism. It wasn't until she was too ill to do it herself that I found out that her ebony color was courtesy of Clairol's Nice 'n Easy. It was perhaps my most unforgettable experience with the parental dictum "Do as I say, not as I do." Without comment I dyed her hair for her a month before she died, and I was sad to see, once she'd lapsed into unconsciousness in the hospital, that her roots were creeping back, the color of steel. The color my hair is turning now.

At first glance I suppose it's still brown, which is what my driver's license says. It's taking its sweet time making the change. In my early forties the grays started to appear, and I did what almost everyone does: I pulled them out. It wasn't simply that they were gray but that they were kind of berserk, *boing boing boing* into some strange awry corkscrews that refused to lie down with the rest. But at a certain point they began to relax, and so did I, and they multiplied, and I had a vision. By fifty my hair would be silver, like the hair of an editor friend who has had a mane of incandescently white hair ever since I first met her. I've always assumed that in her bedroom her hair glows in the dark like a night-light.

That's not what happened to me, although I bought a special

shampoo she recommended that keeps your grays from getting yellow and sternly told the hairdresser that I did not want to have yet another conversation about the healing properties of henna. There was a gray here, a gray there, a swath underneath on one side. People who are really nice, and who like me, say it looks like highlights. I think it looks like dust. But I am glad I followed my mother's advice and didn't start to color it. Between eyebrow waxing, exfoliation, and the occasional laser, I've got all the maintenance I can handle. As far as I know, my mother never exfoliated. Her beauty regimen seemed to consist entirely of Pond's cold cream and Noxzema. Besides, my husband doesn't seem to care about my gray; he only concerns himself with the length of a woman's hair, his motto being "It can never be too long." (His own gray is appearing as though it is being done by the makeup artists for a Broadway production in which the male lead is required to age gracefully between act one and act three. As Bette Davis says about her boyfriend in *All About Eve,* "Bill's thirty-two. He looks thirty-two. He looked it five years ago, he'll look it twenty years from now. I hate men.")

"I wish I could go gray," a woman who works on Wall Street told me. "But that'd be the last straw." It turned out that what she meant was that she'd been overlooked, marginalized, discounted, underestimated, passed over for years, and she couldn't give the guys yet another reason to think she was neglible. That's what changing her hair color from ash blond to ash would have meant to her, and to those around her. It's not just the hair, but the clothes, the makeup, the shoes. One of my closest friends is a fierce dresser, and a fierce competitor, but one day she just got tired of torturing her feet with shoes that are the modern equivalent of the corsets and girdles of yore. She started wearing flats, and she's never turned back. She even wore fancy flip-flops to her daughter's wedding. "She can get away with it because she's so powerful," a younger woman said. In other words, if she was still in the fight she'd better strap on those stilettos, no matter how uncomfortable, to serve notice that she was a coming character, not a has-been.

It's so hard to tell how much of these assumptions are real and how much are our old insecurities wresting away the steering wheel and driving us down a bumpy road even though we're old enough to know better. In her book *Going Gray,* Anne Kreamer decided that the only way she could challenge the working hypothesis—that gray hair inevitably leads to crippled sexual appeal—was to test it. She posted pictures of herself on an Internet dating site, some with brown hair, some with gray. "I assumed, as most might," she wrote, "that men would be more interested in dating the brown-haired me. Well, I couldn't have been more wrong. Turns out three times as many men were interested in going out with me with gray hair."

Bottom line is that none of this is about how we look, but about who we are. No, I'm not preaching the gospel of personality trumping appearance that I absorbed so completely when I was young; if I really believed that, then I've wasted an astonishing amount of money on lipstick and moisturizer.

But I look sometimes at photographs of myself taken over the years, and what's most important, and enduring, transcends my appearance. It is as though I can see not the aging of my face but the story of my life. There is the little girl with the dimples and the authentic and automatic grin. There is the teenager whose eyes are wary, who seems to be worrying about what the camera is seeing. There is the young woman whose mouth smiles but whose eyes do not, the tired young mother too worried about a toddler darting out of the frame to concentrate on her own expression.

And then it is as though I've circled back through time, and the automatic grin has returned. A smile is nature's face-lift, I like to say brightly, now that everything is sliding south. "Let's try a few with a more serious expression," the photographer will say, and I comply, lifting my chin, angling my face, but I know it's the photographs with the smile that I will want. The line of my jaw is sharper, the cheeks fuller. While I eschew the scalpel, I will take cheery and fresh over dour and exhausted any day. And a big smile does that for me.

My dimples are gone, or at least they have been replaced by something else, something less culturally adorable. What were once tiny divots are now deep furrows that stretch almost from cheek to chin. Gains and losses, I think sometimes as I look in the mirror. That's my mantra now: gains and losses. I know more but remember less. My muscles are tight but my skin is loose. I am physically fit but forever infertile. My hair is still thick, but much of it is gray.

When I have my picture taken nowadays, it is most often my daughter who takes it, so the smile always extends to my eyes because it is she behind the camera, smiling back at me and editing as she goes: "Oh, no, that's a bad one, this one I like but you'll hate, *yow,* not that one." In some strange way I feel as though I've resurrected the little girl from my childhood photos, even though her dimply dots have turned to dashes. I don't think she considered for a moment how she appeared in her pictures, and I don't think about it too much anymore. The difference between us is that she thought the world was wonderful, that everyone loved her, and that a tragedy consisted of having the ice cream tumble from her cone onto the hot macadam of the Dairy Queen parking lot. And I, naturally, know different. But she's still in there, thank God, peeking out from time to time, smiling. She's not pretty, that kid, but she has so much pizzazz. Is that me? That's me, I guess.

Solitude

Over the years my household during the summer months has dwindled down to mostly me. In the beginning I piled the kids into the car as soon as school was over and took them out to the country, late June to Labor Day. They went to day camp, messed around in the creek, pumped away on the swings, checked themselves for ticks before they washed off the grime in the tub. But now that they're grown I'm alone in the middle of nowhere, with two dogs and two cats. There are deer, coyote, and fox here, and the occasional bear, but in this part of the world they're scenery. My husband comes out on weekends, but during the week I'm on my own.

There are two different responses to this kind of arrangement. The first is pity, the notion that being alone is synonymous with loneliness and must be remedied with company at all costs. The second is the minority reaction: that solitude sounds wonderful. My closest friend is an only child, and when I first begin this summer idyll—which is nominally for professional reasons, since there is nothing much to do here except write—she always sounds faintly envious. She feels about being alone the way most people feel about chocolate. So does my father, but for a different reason: he was one of eight children.

The second of our three children loves being alone as much as I do. He is so in tune with the satisfaction of solitude that he, too, sometimes comes here alone, or, when I am here, sets himself up to write in his own space in such a way that we intersect, happily, only for meals. He has always been someone whose primary need was to go within to find energy and sustenance.

In the same way that many people assume that being by yourself is an unnatural condition, so when Christopher was young I overlooked or ignored his solitude gene as I buried my own. When he was little, and helpless against my most maniacal mommy impulses, I threw a big party every year for his birthday. Two dozen children and their families would trundle out from the city for a day of hay rides, scavenger hunts, barbecuing, and swimming. They all blur together in my mind now: the year of the Ghostbusters cake, the year of the Jurassic Park cake, squabbles, sunburns, the little boy who erupted in chicken pox during the course of the party and was summarily packed into the car and driven home. They were all the same party, really, and all the same in this: at some point, between the punctured swimmies that needed to be replaced and the tragic frosting in some sensitive little girl's hair, I would realize that Birthday Boy had disappeared. I would almost always find him somewhere out of the way, sleeping, exhausted by the invasion, by the need to be social. If he had been old enough to drive, he would have gotten in the car, cranked up the music, and been out of there. A nap in a back bedroom was the best he could do.

Most of the world finds solitude strange. When I am on my own, I'm importuned with invitations inspired, someone will say, because "You're all by yourself." This is always said in a tone of sadness and concern, except for the occasional fellow traveler who looks at me with an expression that means she would trade places in a heartbeat.

For many years I had virtually no experience of solitude. The oldest of five children, from an extended family as populous as some small towns, I was always one among many. Because my mother had little interest in whether her furniture stayed pristine—with five kids, most of it was in what we like to call earth tones, which is more or less the color of dirt—our house was often the place where other people's children congregated, too. I grew up in a neighborhood that was largely Catholic ("St. Andrew's or St. Bernadette's parish?" someone from the area asked my husband once when he heard where I'd been raised). There were families of seven, eight, nine, even the occasional eleven. There was a girl in my elementary school class who was an object of great curiosity because she had no brothers or sisters. It sounded like an Aesop's fable, the moral being "Be careful what you wish for."

I was truly alone for the first time after college, in a one-bedroom apartment on the top floor of a federal house in lower Manhattan. Even before the children arrived, with their obligatory christenings and birthday parties, I had an odd affinity for labor-intensive social events that sounded better in theory than they were in fact: a ladies' tea for young feminists with home-made scones the consistency of Styrofoam, a Christmas tree–decorating evening at which most of the guests were Jewish (I still have a few of the ornaments they brought along, bless them). But a lot of my time during the years between college and co-habitation was spent by myself, watching miniseries on TV and eating ice cream for dinner with a beer chaser. The reason stereotypes of the haphazard lives of single women exist may be because they're accurate.

My apartment had a fireplace, a wall of windows, and a kitchen the size of my current dining room table; it was what was called charming, which meant it was just the right size for one person who wasn't claustrophobic. I'm not, but even I was frequently driven out into the streets of New York, walking for hours while my winter breath hung in front of me like a ghost leading me on to some glimpse of the future, or the past, or happiness, or conviviality. My memories of those walks are of two related things, lamplight and loneliness, the warm insides of rooms that, in my fantasies, were full of pretty old furniture, lovely pictures, people murmuring to other people about whatever it was that they had to be pleased to be murmuring about. And outside, my fingers numb with cold, me. I had that feeling you have when you're watching a sad movie, sobbing at the heartbreak you are feeling at the same time that you know the heartbreak isn't exactly real, that it will be gone by the time you get home and make a cup of tea. I found a lot of life like that when I was younger, as though I was practicing for what came later.

It seemed very real at the time, though, that introduction to solitude. And it was completely self-inflicted. New York offered parties, events, plays, readings, restaurants. And yet for all of that it can be the loneliest place on earth, far more redolent of isolation than the country place where I maroon myself each summer, silent except for incessant birdsong and the grinding sound from the quarry over the mountain and the faint dribbling noise from the basketball camp up the hill. In the country you are merely alone; in the city you're alone surrounded by thousands of others, close enough to touch, close enough to brush up against, to bump into. When your own solitude is a beating bruise in your chest, it makes it no better to know that on the other side of the kitchen wall is another kitchen, another cook, another person. It makes it worse, like sitting in the obstetrician's office surrounded by big-bellied women when your own is flat and empty.

But that's the involuntary alone. It's something different

when it's freely chosen, and over time I realized that if there were so many opportunities to be in company and I still stayed home, it must mean I liked it. People do confuse alone and lonely, but when you've made the choice to be by yourself, the first has no shadow of the second. Inevitably, age is a time of solitude, not only because at a certain point your friends begin to die—"Last man standing," my father said one day after the news of another passing—but because they, too, become less interested in frantic roundelays of socializing. I remember a time in my life when I gave big dinner parties the way kleptomaniacs steal, and with as little purpose and joy. Boeuf bourguignon, coq au vin, all manner of things that could be made in the big orange Le Creuset pot we got as a wedding gift. Cloth napkins, purposeful seating, bright conversation. I was always so happy when those evenings were over.

Sometimes, for some of us, being sociable is a tyranny, a function of custom, society, peer pressure, sheer youthful craziness. I gave those dinners at the flip-up table in my single-girl apartment, invited all those third-graders to run ragged through our country house, put on the shoes and the mascara and got in the cab for cocktails, to send a message to the world: this is the sort of person I am. Only I wasn't, not really.

When one of my children was being tested for attention deficit disorder—and I was answering yes in my mind to all the questions the therapist asked—it occurred to me that perhaps I had a mind that was easily overloaded, that needed to wipe itself clean with some regularity. Maybe I'm hardwired to want to spend time alone; I remember a childhood reading books in the living room while my friends were playing street games just outside. Or maybe it's a function of my chaotic upbringing. Eldest children are often much more understanding of the need to be alone; I am an eldest child, as is my husband, a marriage of two executive-function humans that I sometimes joke should be outlawed by Congress. ("The eldest child of two eldest children": that is how our son once described himself, which I believe was subtle shorthand for "heat-seeking missile.") As a group we are actually rather good at being alone in a crowd, like that old film construct in which the spirit climbs out of a character and comments on the scene. We're there but not there, social, smiling, but somehow somewhere else.

Or maybe my yearning to be by myself is a function of my life as a novelist, the need to go within to create an imaginary world, although when I think of all those stories about hard-partying writers, about Hemingway and Mailer and Capote, I know that not all writers need or can even tolerate solitude. (Come to think of it, the female of the species seems more inclined: think Jane Austen, Flannery O'Connor, Eudora Welty, the Brontës.) I've stopped trying to figure out why I do what I do, which is another gift of late maturity: I fear heights, love liver and onions, prefer big dogs to small ones, work best between the hours of ten and two. Who knows why? Who cares? I prize my downtime, count on it as a writer, a parent, a person. Sometimes I think of Woody Allen's remark about masturbation, that it is sex with someone he loves. I feel as though being alone is hanging out with someone I like.

Luckily I'm not alone. One of my friends came to our house in the country one weekend and, after breakfast, disappeared into her room or into the woods with a book. She showed up for lunch, disappeared again, then showed up showered and dressed to help with dinner, have a drink, talk, as the evening lowered and then came down like a Roman shade of soft summer night. I wasn't worried a bit, but my husband, who is a more social animal than I am, pulled me aside to say, "I'm afraid Jean isn't having a good time. She keeps going off by herself."

"She's fine," I said. "She's perfect." She was.

When I was young I was loath to admit that I liked being alone, but not anymore. By the time you've lived for fifty or sixty years, you are better armored to embrace the things about yourself that are true, even if you might think the world sees them as odd, eccentric. I have a much greater tolerance for ambiguity now. Human progress on both a political and a personal level means dicta are always a moving target: God Save the King gives way to All Men Are Created Equal, Always Wear Hose is blessedly retired in favor of Whatever Gets You Through the Night. I remember learning the Baltimore Catechism word for word, mainly because along with spelling bees we had catechism bees, and I'm your girl if you're looking for some competition. "Why did God make me? To know him, to love him, and to serve him in this world, and to be happy with him forever in the next." Trust me, that's the right answer. To something. Although not to something to which I've been able to subscribe for the last thirty years of my life.

There are a few eternal verities, and many of them are rock songs: love is often all you need, you can't always get what you want, and the new boss is indeed the same as the old boss. But so much of what we say and do is empty. I remember one afternoon when our elder son made this clear to me. It was second semester of his junior year in high school, a time that for a smart, directed boy is akin to being locked in a room with a hive of angry bees. And he just got tired of being stung. "I want to know the point of all this!" he yelled. "I worked hard in grade school so I could go to a good high school, and I'm working hard in high school so I can get into a good college. And after that, what's the point? A good job, right? And then? And then? What's the endgame?"

"Oh, honey," I said, lapsing into the pat answer we absorb in the kind of obsessive miasma of free-floating worry we call parenting. "Your dad and I just want you to be happy." And with that he slammed his hand down on the dining room table so hard I jumped in my seat, and shouted, "Mom, none of this has anything to do with being *happy*!"

When I was young I wasn't bright or brave enough to ask

that sort of question, just wanted to get things settled, although it often turned out that I had no idea what that meant. I saw a boy across a crowded room in college and decided to marry him with no thought about how long marriage was, and how challenging. I nailed down a profession and pursued it single-mindedly. In my early twenties I asked my doctor to tie my tubes so that I would never have children; to his credit, he stubbed out his omnipresent cigarette—a doctor who smoked: now, there's a marker of age—and said he'd be happy to discuss this if I saw a therapist to thoroughly talk over my reasons. (My reasons were simple, and understandable: my siblings were motherless, I had been cast in the role of reluctant caregiver, I didn't like it, they didn't like it. Later there would be many made-for-television movies on this and related topics.) A decade later, with no sense of the inherent irony, I suddenly decided I wanted a baby immediately, and that time no doctor stopped me, and there was a baby, then another, and another.

But of course it's not that things get settled, as though life was a résumé or a checklist: husband, children, work. "Life is what happens to you while you're busy making other plans," as John Lennon famously said. It's taken me years, not to understand that intellectually but to internalize it emotionally, which eventually leads to the "one day at a time" approach, favored by 12-step addiction programs, applied to your actual life. It's one of the best parts of growing up and growing older, I think, that feeling that you'll just get through one day, and then the next, that a week from Saturday will take care of itself. I couldn't do that when I was younger.

I don't know how much of this knowledge grows out of being female and having lived through layers of serial, often contradictory, lives. We women spend our whole lives going up and down hormonally, being one thing on Wednesday and another on Sunday, feeling bloated and then svelte, juicy and then played out. And our bodies have changed so often during our lifetimes—puberty, pregnancy, menopause, premenstrual, post-menstrual, posthysterectomy, sometimes postmastectomy—that having a different body than we had at thirty comes as less of a surprise to us than it does to many men. From the time they reach puberty, boys are, let's be honest, sex bombs who live it 24/7. They tie much of their self-image to their potency and wind up, over their life spans, making an awful lot of remarks in an awful lot of settings about whose is bigger, both literally and metaphorically. The loss of that potency slowly but surely diminishes them in their own minds, while many women find the loss of fertility a relief, particularly if they've had a few kids.

It's hard to communicate to our male counterparts that one of the greatest gifts of growing older is trusting your own sense of yourself; their investment in their reflected image was not forged in childhood, as ours was. Sometimes I think women, freed from societal expectations and roles, age into confidence, while men, losing the power, status, and strength of youth, age out of it. All I really know about myself is what the big rock outside my writing porch has engraved on it: "Nothing is written in stone."

For years I lived every day devoted to the welfare of three exuberant, emotionally exhausting children. Because of what he did, their father went off to the office every day, where he lived a life separate from Chicken McNuggets, sticky surfaces, late-afternoon meltdowns, and the need to find graph paper and a compass *right now.* Because of what I do, I stayed at home. I envied Gerry the solitude of the car, the office, the bathroom break not interrupted by questions through the closed door or shrieks from the next room.

I don't subscribe to the jokey dictum that retirement comes when the last child leaves home and the dog dies. I love being with my kids, and so does their father, and I expect that there will be dogs in perpetuity. Actually, I like solitude with dogs. You can hear someone else breathing, but you don't feel obliged to tell them about your day, or to hear about their own, or to share the brownie batter bowl. You can't do that with your children, can't say, "Honey, Mommy had four younger siblings and she never got the brownie bowl all to herself, and now she really, really wants it. Alone. With a big wooden spoon."

Being alone is not the same as being on your own, but it's related to it. That's something that women are supposed to hate and fear—the responsibility for the life insurance, the heating oil delivery, the dripping faucet, the car inspections. Or there is the greater fear, what is sometimes called bag lady syndrome, the terror that as the years go by the money will run out. Even prosperous women have it, and with good reason—a substantial percentage of those living below the poverty line are women in their later years. Sometimes we look at the amount in the pension plan, the retirement account, the investment portfolio, and do calculations that scare us. With longer life comes the need for a larger safety net, and we fear the holes in that net.

I suppose we older women have more reason to fear being alone than our male counterparts. Often we've made less money and more concessions. The great whispered story of too many marriages is that he left her for a younger woman. (And, by the way, if you happen to be one of those men, please spare me the rhapsodies about how you're available for your second clutch of kids as you weren't for your first.) The great public tragedy of many of those marriages is that he died first, leaving her without a lifelong partner. Our children start families of their own, families that take precedence and that sometimes take them far away, with only time for the occasional visit, and what it comes down to eventually is one woman living in a house too big for her. It can't be good for her, being all by herself, can it?

But sometimes I think that in this, as in so much else, we tend to sell women short. I go to a funeral for a friend's father, and she whispers that she doesn't know how her mother will get along, that she moved directly from her parents' house into the one she shared with her husband, that she's never written a check or paid a bill. Her children are swooping in to take charge, to take over, so that now the woman in the corner, with her coiffed hair and nude hose and black knit dress, will become their dependent. But months later, I ask about Mom and am told, with a note of surprise and just a suggestion of suspicion, "She seems to be doing really well." She's taking a trip. She's joined a book club. She's selling the house. She's learned to pay bills. She's on her own. It is a terrifying thought, not dinner for one but life for one, too. It is a terrifying thought, and sometimes, for a woman who has always been surrounded by others, a liberating thought as well. There is so much obligatory generosity to being a good mother, a good wife, a good friend. Solitude is an acceptable form of selfishness.

PART III

The Element of Surprise

How old would you be if you didn't know how old you were?
—SATCHEL PAIGE

Every once in a while we meet our long-ago selves across a dining table or a desk, when younger women come to ask for advice or to interview for a job. They're so eager and so smart, with their dresses and their shiny hair, and we know exactly what they want because we once wanted it, too. They want a formula, a plan, a set of directions, an assembly kit. Connect A to B, C to D, and in the end there it is, the life you crave. The job, the salary, the companion, the home.

It's so hard to tell them the truth, that there is no formula, no plan. It's harder still to communicate that your life has been filled with accidents and that they have determined so much of how things turned out. Some have been happy accidents, some not. There were plans for a family but the right partner didn't come along, or came along too late. There were plans for a big family but after the first child there was no other, or plans for an only child that were changed by an accidental pregnancy. My early plans to have no children at all morphed into plans to have four, and we wound up with three. And now that seems exactly right, even fated somehow. It's amazing how resilient people are, and how the things that didn't come true become, after a while, simply the way things are.

It often seems, looking back, that the unexpected comes to define us, the paths we didn't see coming and may have wandered down by mistake. The older we get the more willing we are to follow those, to surprise ourselves. After all, all we can do is fail, and failure loses so much of its sting over time. We not only know how to fall, we know how to get up. We've done it so often.

Failure is so terrifying to the young. So is unpredictability. They're afraid they'll get it wrong. You have to use cookbooks for a long time before you realize that you can leave out the beans, throw in some tomatoes, substitute rosemary for basil, jettison the formula, try something different. Sometimes the improvisation is better than the original recipe, sometimes just as good, and sometimes you pour it down the Disposall and make a nice fettucine Alfredo, which never hurt anyone.

Eleanor Roosevelt once famously said that it was important to do something every day that scared you, and it's a pretty good piece of advice. But it's more challenging when you're older because you're afraid of fewer things, certainly fewer of those small everyday things that I think Eleanor meant. The things we fear now supplant asking for a raise or sending a story to a magazine or inviting a stranger to dinner. They are more cosmic, more philosophical, about a more difficult and dependent future. Perhaps instead of scaring ourselves we need to surprise ourselves every day. We are, after all, always a work in progress. There were things I hadn't done, didn't know, couldn't imagine at fifty that have all come true in the last decade. There must be such things in the decades to come as well. They arrive not because of the engraved invitations of careful planning but through happy happenstance, doodles on the to-do list of life.

The Little Stories We Tell Ourselves

This is a story about balance, strength, and persistence. It's about the determination not to give up and give in, the refusal to see "older" as synonymous with "less." And at the end I stand on my head.

It took me two years to get there, but today I can do a headstand at a moment's notice. No brag, just fact. Actually, it's all brag. I worked hard on this headstand, indefatigably, systematically, harder than I've worked on my own work, which comes fairly naturally to me. What I don't have naturally is a sense of balance.

"That's just a little story you tell yourself," said Anita, who is a trainer, performs weddings, makes jewelry, and functions as a kind of freelance Italian American guru.

Oh, those little stories we tell ourselves. They make us what we are, and, too often, what we're not. They are the ten commandments of incapability, cut to order. I can't cook. I'm not smart. I'm a bad driver. I'm no jock. Maybe they're even true.

It's hard to tell at a certain point. The little stories we tell ourselves become mythic, difficult if not impossible to discount or overcome. They get written into our DNA, so that when the plane hits a bump, adrenaline floods our bodies as we say to ourselves, "I am afraid of flying." Sometimes over time it becomes clear how many of the little stories are fictional or, more particularly, lies.

As we age there are the stories we tell ourselves about our lack of allure, our physical incapacity, even our degeneration. So far my body has not betrayed me with illness or infirmity, but I am always watching, especially on what I think of as Mortality Mondays, when I have my annual mammogram first thing on a fall morning. All we have to do is look at the data to know that our suspicions of our very own self as incubus have some foundation, that something bad may be happening within even as we eat our leafy greens, walk briskly up the stairs, take the multivitamin. The price we pay for an information culture is that every day, in every way, we are learning that our bodies could let us down.

Let's face it: they already have. We may have more equanimity about how we look, but we've managed to achieve that equanimity just at the moment when our bodies are starting to be less, not by twisted cultural standards but by the standards of our own past lives. When I was young I was voluble about the shortcomings of my legs (bowed), my breasts (large), my butt (ditto), my waist (nonexistent). It almost goes without saying that I looked fine. Now I'm mainly running to stay in place, and when I do, sometimes something hurts. It's just the way things are, but it doesn't mean we have to like it, or even accept it.

We each find the thing about these inevitable changes that makes us crazy. For me it happens to be my eyes. I'm short-waisted and flat-footed, but I've always had perfect vision. I was the person who could read the fine print on the container of children's Tylenol, spot the street sign a block away from a moving car, thread a needle without scrunching up my face.

Ah, but that was then. This is now. I have glasses. Many pairs of glasses. I have so many because they are somehow never where I am. The red ones, the tortoiseshell ones. I wander the house and find three pairs in my purse, although not the purse I am currently using. "Here they are," I am always saying.

The optometrist was so jolly when I bought the first pair. How old? Forty-two. Right on schedule, he crowed. You know what they say, he said. It's not that your vision's bad, it's that your arms are too short. Magnification 1.75, then 2.25, now 3.0. I hate my glasses because they were the very first thing that alerted me to the notion that I was on a slippery slope of losing—my hair color, my jawline, my bone mass, my vision. I keep a magnifying mirror on the vanity in the bathroom even though I believe it's a tool of the devil.

My memory, too, has become a strange shape-shifter, playing hide-and-seek with the obvious. I lose a number or a name for fifteen or twenty minutes and then it returns, so indelible that I can't quite understand how it was ever gone. Word retrieval is a bit of a challenge, which would be less important if I didn't have to build a house of sentences almost every day. Conspicuous. Perfunctory. Malfeasance. They hang in the air somewhere to the left of my conscious brain, where my mind could pick them up if my mind had peripheral vision. I can feel the shape of them, the syllables, usually the first letter. Then, like the Cheshire cat, they materialize while I'm not paying attention and I slam them into print so they can't disappear again.

Which would we rather, this or the more physical, the aching back, the wonky hip? Neither, thank you.

When we were kids we used to amuse ourselves with physical disasters that never happened. If you had to choose, would you be blind or deaf? (Deaf.) If you had to lose an arm or a leg, which would it be? (Arm. Everyone said arm.) But of course, being young, we never asked ourselves the questions that now concern or haunt us, the real questions: Is that pain between the eyes a hangover, a headache, or a brain tumor?

The way the human body works, or, finally, doesn't, reminds me of a run-in I had with a Cuisinart full of the ingredients for black bean soup. I turned the lid and instead of the familiar growl heard nothing but silence. Again. Again. Rattled it, the last refuge of the angry nonmechanically minded. Gave it a shot of WD-40 and tried not to think what that was going to do to the taste of the soup. Then finally said aloud, "I can't believe this damn thing conked out after only"—and did the math in my head, then did it again. The Cuisinart had been a wedding gift, which meant that I had been using it for more than thirty years. After all that time I should have delivered an impassioned eulogy for the thing instead of hitting it with a spatula.

Our bodies, too, are major appliances that have delivered decades of faithful service with precious little downtime. I've been bending these knees since they were scabby and scraped from falling on the pavement, been walking on these flat feet since I was ten months old, been using these eyes for six decades. If the human body had a warranty, mine would have run out ages ago.

It's indisputable that I'm not the newer model. There's an Agatha Christie novel in which a major plot fulcrum has to do with the knees of one of the characters. She's been pretending to be quite a young woman, but she's actually considerably older, and our ace detective knows this by looking at her knees. I can't remember whether the detective is Miss Marple or Hercule Poirot, or even what the story was about; one of the great things about being the age I am now and having a reliably unreliable memory is that I can reread mystery novels. I either don't remember whodunit or, when I do figure it out, I convince myself that it's because I'm canny and wise. All I can remember about that particular book is the knees. And because of it, from time to time, I have looked at my own, squinting suspiciously. I can't compare them to my knees at twenty; I never paid the least bit of attention to my knees at twenty. But I'm quite certain they had something that they don't have now. Everything tells me so.

One of the reasons I passed quietly into the country of menopause is, I think, that I had an adolescent girl around the house whose estrogen was in hyperdrive at the same time my own gauge was inching toward empty. There are lots of advantages to having children in your thirties instead of your twenties—for me, it meant that I never looked down at a sleeping infant and thought, Darn it, wish I was out clubbing—but one is that it eventually makes it impossible for you to deny that hormones are a dangerous controlled substance. When your daughter enters the house, throws her backpack across the dining room, stomps up the stairs, and slams her bedroom door with a sound like a building being dynamited, then screams, "Nothing!" when you ask what's wrong, there's a temptation to think that she's overreacting. But not if you've woken in a cold sweat at 2:00 A.M., incapable of finding sleep again, staring at a crack in the moonlit ceiling and thinking about how your husband's regular breathing makes you want to elbow him, hard. Unless you're completely unhinged—and some of the time that may be the case—you can't help realizing that you and your daughter are having different variations on the same theme. She up, you down. She in, you out.

Modern medicine has made it possible for women to pretend that their fecund years are not over, by providing hormones that come out of pill vials instead of ovaries. These were originally sold as something to keep us cheerful so we wouldn't annoy men. One early ad for Premarin featured a photograph of an adoring woman watching a man pilot a boat, with the accompanying words, "It is no easy thing for man to take the stings and barbs of business life, then to come home to the turmoil of a woman 'going through the change of life.'" (Unfortunately the next frame of the ad does not show the woman smashing a hole in the bottom of the boat, allowing it to fill with water and then sink.)

People today discuss hormones as a fountain of youth for everything from the bones to the skin to the memory; in other words, at a time of systematic losing, you can be a winner through chemistry. I've had friends who swear that that kind of pharmaceutical intervention saved their lives, saved them from mood swings so severe that they felt like a multiple personality case on a bad day. Luckily I was spared the worst; I mostly wound up taking the sweater off and putting the sweater on, so I took a pass on the pills and the patch for any number of reasons. Perhaps because my mother took a synthetic estrogen called DES during her pregnancies that cost me long diagnostic hours in doctors' offices, I'm someone who responds to the directive "Take this" with the question "Why?"

But eschewing hormones doesn't mean I don't want to find my own fountain of youth, or at least fountain of youthful. There was nothing I could do about my eyes except wear glasses, and I'm not sure any of those skin creams make a bit of difference. Instead I decided that rather than hold on to what I'd once had, I would find some way to become something new. My doctor, who is about the same age as I am, provided a way to make that happen at just about the same time that my vision started to blur. On a prescription pad she wrote, "Hire a trainer."

(It's interesting how much force a scrip gives to a simple directive. A friend told me her husband, a psychiatrist, once wrote two for a patient, one for a mild antidepressant and another that said, "Get a dog." The guy got a dog, too, and I'm going to guess that that was at least as much help in mood elevation as the pills.)

Those trainers—Jenny, Anita, Meegan, I salute you—led me to dead lifts and one-legged squats and biceps curls. They led me to question the little stories I'd long told myself about my strength and my balance, and that led me to the headstand, my personal symbol of opposition to the pernicious pessimism that accompanies aging. There's something seductive about the thing we believe we cannot do, the achievement that seems out of reach. I imagine it's what keeps people climbing mountains or surfing during storms, that sense of going to the edge of possibility and then over it successfully.

I've never been that kind of risk taker. I avoided physical derring-do, especially anything that required me to take my feet off the ground. The fact that all three of my children wanted to go skydiving made me wonder whether they'd been switched at birth. But as I assessed the bill of goods I'd sold myself over the decades, it occurred to me that maybe I'd reached a moment when I could stop telling myself old stories and start inventing some new ones.

Part of it was sheer stubbornness, the notion that I will accept the things I cannot change but will change the things I can or die trying. Isaac Newton learned about gravity from a falling apple; I learned about gravity from my butt, and I'm fighting the falling. Hence the free weights, the kettle bells, the Swiss ball, the Bosu ball, the medicine balls, and the weighted balls. One day my husband looked around our bedroom and said, "Are you making a model of the solar system?" Pilates teaser, triceps dips, torso twists: sometimes it all makes me a little sad. If I'd worked out like this when I was twenty-five, I would have been a goddess. Except that I wouldn't have worked out like this when I was twenty-five. There is, I'm convinced, a kind of dogged determination that can come with getting older, a determination not to be overcome by can't or don't, by perceived shortcomings. I feel it most conspicuously when I work out. Chest press . . . *I will not* . . . side plank . . . *let myself* . . . squat thrust . . . *be beaten.* Push-up push-up push-up. Crunch crunch crunch.

I would have sworn to you when I was younger that I would never have wound up here on the bedroom floor, huffing and puffing and pumping iron. The little story I told myself then was that I wasn't the kind of woman who exercised. I have a short attention span, and I'd always rather run my mouth than run. I haven't since become one of those exercise junkies, buzzing on endorphins and sweat. But I've finally recognized my body for what it is: a personality delivery system, designed expressly to carry my character from place to place, now and in the years to come. It's like a car, and while I like a red convertible or even a Bentley as well as the next person, what I really need are four tires and an engine. I don't require a hood ornament. It's not about how my body looks at this point; it's about how it works.

We women have such a strange relationship with our bodies nowadays, even stranger than it was when I was a girl. All of it takes place at the margins, between the Boston Marathon and all-you-can-eat buffets, between draconian diet plans and the Triple Quarter Pounder with cheese. Obesity and anorexia—you have to hand it to us Americans, we never do anything halfway. We have a culture that elevates women in advertisements who are contoured like thirteen-year-old boys, a culture that showcases actresses on television so undernourished that they look like bobblehead dolls. We've invented a new—and apparently desirable—class of clothes, size 0. A Harvard University study showed that up to two-thirds of underweight twelve-year-old girls considered themselves to be too fat. In other words, we have a culture that reflects contempt and antipathy toward a realistic female body, which is just another form of hating women.

That's *not* a little story we tell ourselves. It's a story everything around us tells us, and, worse, it's a story young women hear as they're growing to adulthood. The invisible negligible disappearing woman, the cultural ideal just at a time when women are becoming more powerful and participatory in the world. No mystery to that equation. And speaking of equations, zero is nothing.

I will never be skinny. I want to be strong, strong enough to hike the mountain across the road without getting breathless, strong enough to take a case of wine from the deliveryman and carry it to the kitchen. Strong enough to physically fight the weak-woman surrender that I've been fighting spiritually all my life; when I work out hard enough I feel like I want to go out and knock over a convenience store, and for a woman who grew up with her hands folded and her knees together, that's one fabulous feeling. Scarlett O'Hara had a seventeen-inch waist, but she couldn't eat anything at the barbecue, and at the end of the book she's alone. What's so great about that? When I was first challenged to do the headstand and insisted I was too old to learn a new trick, someone told me that story about a fifty-year-old woman who says she can't get a college degree at her age. "By the time I'm done I'll be fifty-four," she tells a friend, and her friend replies, "In four years you'll be fifty-four anyway."

Maybe I also decided to do the headstand because I was afraid to do it, and I don't like the idea that I'm afraid. My father was a management consultant, and he taught me about W. Edwards Deming, the business guru who is best known for the reconstruction of the Japanese economy after World War II. Deming has a list of managerial dicta, and one of them is "Drive out fear." It's an essential part of maturing, putting fear aside, because if there's anything that cripples us it is fear. In some ways I think it's the essential evil because it is the root of so many others. We don't take jobs we would love because we are afraid to try something new. We don't move to another city or end a bad relationship because fear smothers adventure and self-interest. We hate new immigrants, people of different back-grounds and races, those with opposing views, because we are afraid, afraid to find out that we are not special, chosen, dominant, right. All great despots play on the fear of their people to get them to embrace bigotry and xenophobia. When you look back on the evil we've done as a country or the chances we've missed as individuals, fear is almost always the driving force. When we were girls, many of us feared being ourselves.

As I like to tell students who believe that if you do something competently you must enjoy it, I hate to write precisely because I am afraid every time I look at a blank computer screen, afraid of the gap between what I imagine and what actually materializes. My father declared after his eightieth birthday that he was now part of the Eighty Plus Club and that its members had different rules than do the rest of us. Most of them seemed to consist of not doing things my father didn't want to do. As a member of the fifty-plus crowd I'm not getting on a roller coaster or even a Tilt-A-Whirl. I reserve the right to certain insignificant aversions.

I was afraid of the headstand, afraid to be upside down in a way that had a lot more to do with fear than with balance. But nailing it was about fear, too, about being able to will agility and ability into being at a time when so much told me that I was aging out of both. And I had to understand and analyze both my strengths and weaknesses to do so. I wasted a year trying to do a headstand the way the flexible yoga types do, just springing up and over. I'm not flexible, physically or spiritually, and it was when I decided to use my strength and determination instead that I got where I wanted to go. Tripod, leg raise, pelvic tilt. And one day I was up, and then upside down. The world didn't look much different except that it turned out there was a lot of spare change and a couple of stray earrings under my bureau. But it felt different. I can do something today that I couldn't do half a century ago. And if I can do one thing like that, perhaps there are others. The learning curve continues, which is just another way of saying you're alive.

This isn't one of those parables about how everything is possible. We do our children a disservice with the new fashion of suggesting that's so: "You can do anything you set your mind to" is a lovely sentiment, but it's a bait and switch for the kid with a mediocre voice who sets his sights on Broadway. But sometimes I look at my own existence and think of how improbable most of it is: How I came to live in the city that seems to suit my metabolism the way hot fudge suits vanilla ice cream. How I wound up with three children when I once thought I wanted none at all. How I ached to write novels and managed to do so. I know that along the way I told myself a little story about every stop, a story that always contained the word *can't*. But one day, reporter that I am, I decided not to write the story in advance of the facts. I'm focusing on one-armed push-ups at the moment; I suppose they're good for the chest and back, but that has nothing to do with why I want to do them. They're the kind of thing a woman my age can't expect of herself. That's just another little story, and I'm refusing to tell it. Right now I can do three one-armed push-ups on each side. But a year from now, who knows? Who knows?

Older

Here's what happens when you raise the question of getting older at a restaurant table or a cocktail party or standing in line at a coffee shop: the moans begin, the sighs, the eye rolling. John had a hip replacement. Jane has tennis elbow. The back hurts, the feet ache. And let's not even talk about age spots or eyesight or buying a bathing suit.

But what I've found is that if you push people a little harder, ask them what's so terrible about getting older, almost everyone eventually gets past the plantar fasciitis and the crepey neck and winds up admitting that they're happier now than they were when they were young. They feel as if they've settled into their own skin, even if that skin has sun damage.

A Gallup poll of 340,000 people showed unequivocally that we get more contented as we age. Respondents started out at eighteen feeling really good about themselves and their lives, then became less and less satisfied as the years went by. But after age fifty there was a change in the weather, and from then on happiness was on an upward trajectory into the eighties. As those in the survey grew older, they reported that stress, anger, sadness all declined. Perhaps if we think of life as a job, most of us finally feel that after fifty we've gotten good at it.

All this reminds me of a system I once learned to help make any important decision. Take a sheet of paper, draw a line down the middle, list pros and cons. The old house has a leaky roof, rattling windows, a wilderness of a garden, a damp basement, bad gutters. All cons. I love the place. One pro that obliterates all the others.

We can graph good sense all we want, but most of the time we feel what we feel. We can lay out the downside with ease. Getting older means the disintegration of the body, and sometimes the mind. It means being seen as yesterday's news. Perhaps because I grew up in the newspaper business I always realized someday I'd be yesterday's news. Perhaps because I'm the oldest of five, I've always felt older. There's a lot less to my future than there is to my past, and there are undoubted minefields along the way. But what can I tell you? I look at the list of pros and cons, and I always come to the same conclusion. I like the house.

This feeling goes double for women, and the reasons are clear when you talk to them. We started out pretending, trying to adjust our throttle to some generally accepted notion of femininity. In her commencement address to the graduating class of Barnard College in 2010, Meryl Streep said that the characterization of the pleasing girl she created in high school was a role she worked on harder than any ever after. Speaking for so many of us, she recalled, "I adjusted my natural temperament, which tends to be slightly bossy, a little opinionated, a little loud, full of pronouncements and high spirits, and I willfully cultivated softness, agreeableness, a breezy natural sort of sweetness, even shyness if you will, which was very, very, very effective on the boys." Gloria Steinem coined the term "female impersonators" to describe the uncomfortable way in which we women learned early on to play the role of pleaser, with a practiced smile that did not always extend to our eyes.

The act took its toll, as subterfuge and self-denial tend to do, and we paid with an internal dialogue of criticism. Not smart enough, not pretty enough, not a good enough mother, not a good enough professional. An entire Greek chorus chimed in, a Greek chorus made up of magazines, movies, advice books, alleged friends, and family members who insisted they were telling us only for our own good, only wanted to be certain we would be happy and have no regrets. The problem was, the chorus couldn't make up its mind; the messages ranged from self-sacrifice to self-promotion, abstinence to sexual freedom. The only constant was that somehow we all needed to be more than we already were, even if that meant playing a role that was essentially false. But more was never enough. Put together all the mixed messages and what you came up with was an ideal woman who was the six-foot swizzle stick in fashion magazines grafted onto a Supreme Court justice, with three successful children and a husband who loved to cook. Notice that there is no one on earth who conforms to this description.

The only good thing you can say about this nonsense is that at a certain age we learned to see right through it, and that age is now.

Without the aid of self-help books or inspirational speeches, we came to understand that we look and live fine. By the standards that matter, of friendship and diligence and support and loyalty, we are scoring in the top stanine. Cellulite is not a character defect. At sixty you can look all the superwoman stuff in the face and say to yourself, oh, puh-leeze. The Greek chorus is just faint hurdy-gurdy music in the back of your mind on a bad day.

Of course, men have not had to deal with these same expectations or demands. The world still permits them to live relatively unexamined lives in terms of how to see themselves;

when's the last time you saw the headline "Five Pounds in Five Days!" on the cover of *Esquire*? In some fashion this actually makes aging more challenging for men. The constant loop of self-criticism doesn't end when they are older; it begins there. They wake up at sixty and find themselves flabbergasted if they're not masters of the universe. By contrast, the women of our generation have usually found themselves a bit surprised at reaching a high rung on the ladder, which is why we talk about luck so often when we talk about accomplishment.

The result is that many, if not most, women embrace their later years, although they don't know exactly how to name them. Age is just a number, one saying goes, and like most sayings it has a pleasing sound and means exactly nothing. Age is experience, and arthritis, and receding gums, and old stories, and old friends, and presbyopia, and hot flashes. But what is "old"? What does the word mean at a moment when seventy-year-olds run marathons and corporations, have children (well, the guys anyhow), and appear in movies as the leads and not only the character parts? Is it the first time a clerk calls you ma'am instead of miss? Yeah, you remember that moment, stock-still in your Capri pants, with your big sunglasses pushed up into your salon–sun-streaked hair. How about when the girl behind the glass at the movie theater asks if you want a senior citizen's ticket, or when the first mailing comes from AARP? Or, conversely, there's that moment when someone at a bar or liquor store cards you—because it's their policy to card everyone—and your heart soars, or when your dentist tells you you have the gums of a thirty-year-old and it's the high point of your day.

Or maybe it's when you're driving along the thruway with an old, old friend, someone with whom you've shared job struggles and romantic travails and too much tequila and maybe a joint or two, and you find yourself discussing the fact that neither of you is as comfortable driving at night as you once were.

"This is old-people talk," you say, and he replies, "As Bob Dylan once said, he who is not busy being born is busy dying." I wonder which one Dylan thought he was, once he'd moved past the formerly statutory retirement age of sixty-five?

We can all do simple math, yet realizing you've become a person of a certain age comes on suddenly, an incongruous surprise. It came to me full force on a muggy day in July, when a tornado struck our house in Pennsylvania. The dogs pressed against the back of my legs as I made a sandwich in the kitchen, apparently sensing something coming several minutes before I did. Then the wind roared through with a freight-train sound, and the trees bowed down outside the window. In an instant the trees had disappeared, obscured by thick gray air flecked with black, like ominous confetti. In the time it took to assemble lunch, it was, then was not. All that was left was the afterward. Most of the big trees closest to the house were gone, their root balls upended into the air, as though the hand of God had wiped the landscape and ordered us to try again. The pond was filled with downed cedars and enormous willow branches. There was no power and no water, but the house was untouched except for a single cracked chimney cap.

I sent all three of the children messages. Chris was at a German heavy metal festival and didn't get his for days. Quin was in the New York apartment and wrote back immediately, concerned about whether he should come posthaste. But Maria left her university summer school class early and called, sobbing.

"I'm just afraid of history repeating itself," said my daughter, who knows that my own mother died when I was still in college.

And without thinking I responded, "Oh, honey, I'm too old to die young now."

Sometimes things pop out of your mouth that amount to an epiphany, even if they sound like bad country-western songs. This was one of those things. I am no longer young and certainly not elderly. I am past the midpoint of my life. I am at a good point in my life.

Am I old? Define your terms. One afternoon I went a little ballistic when I read a newspaper story that described an "elderly couple" fending off a burglar. The woman involved was sixty-eight. "How is that elderly?" I ranted. "That's not elderly! Sixty-eight is not elderly!"

After the rant, silence, and then one of my children said, "Mom, that's elderly."

"It is," said another.

"Definitely," said the third.

Nonsense, I thought, and to prove it I went to various journalism sites and writing style books to nail down the cutoff point for "elderly," the precise definition of an old person, or an older one. It seems that old is a moving target. Some gerontologists divide us into the young-old, ages fifty-five to seventy-four, and the old-old, over seventy-five. In a survey done by the Pew Research Center, most people said old age begins at sixty-eight. But most people over the age of sixty-five thought it began at seventy-five.

When I searched my own clippings over the course of a long career in journalism for the word "elderly," I discovered to my horror that I had used the adjective with casual regularity. There were the elderly men on the boardwalk in Coney Island, the elderly women in the beauty parlors of Flatbush. And then—here's the important thing—the number of uses of the word "elderly" in my copy began to dwindle, and then they died. As I aged, "elderly" seemed more and more pejorative, and my definition of what constituted elderly shifted upward.

In other words, old is wherever you haven't gotten to yet.

It's all relative, the way it was when I got pregnant for the first time at thirty-one and everyone in our two families thought I'd left it rather late and everyone in our urban friendship circle thought I was rushing into it. When I mentioned writing about aging, women in their seventies and eighties brushed me off: "Oh, you're too young to write about the subject." The truth is, I feel young. I certainly feel a good deal younger than the older people of my past. Our grandmothers at sixty, and my friends and I at the same age: we might as well be talking about different species, in the way we dress, talk, work, exercise, plan—in the way we live. When people lived to sixty-five, sixty *was* old. When they live to be eighty, sixty is something else. We're just not sure what yet. A friend told me she thought it was summed up in the message inside a birthday card she got from her mother: "After the middle ages comes the renaissance."

So we face an entirely new stage of human existence without nomenclature, which is an interesting challenge, because what we call things matters. That's why I recoiled from "elderly." The words we use, and how we perceive those words, reflect how we value, or devalue, people, places, and things. After all, one of the signal semantic goals of the early women's movement was to make certain grown women were no longer referred to as "girls."

I'm also keenly aware of this because I am a writer and I know each word denotes something singular; that's why I was Anna Quindlen before I married and Anna Quindlen afterward, too, because the words "Anna Quindlen" mean a specific person, and that person is me.

Or perhaps one of the reasons I absorbed the importance of naming lies in my childhood. On my upper lip, to one side of center, I have a noticeable raised brown spot, and when I was a little girl my mother taught me that it was something called a beauty mark. In fact, on Halloween, if I were dressed as someone dishy, a gypsy or a princess or a ballerina, my mother would add more beauty marks with a black eyebrow pencil, on one cheek, at the corner of my eye. From time to time my mother would point out beautiful actresses who had beauty marks, too; she thought Elizabeth Taylor was the most gorgeous woman in the world, and Elizabeth Taylor had a beauty mark. The words my mother had used to describe what was on my face had made me completely comfortable with it. I often wondered afterward whether I would have felt otherwise had she said that what was on my face was a mole, which is what it is.

It's too late to rehabilitate the words "old" and "elderly," especially in this age of perpetual youth, so we've redefined them, often redefined them out of existence. We don't even have a name for this time of our lives, or a name that seems to work. Second adulthood, one writer called it. The third chapter, says another. Late middle age? Later age?

Sixty is the new forty, as I'm sure you've heard. And you're only as young as you feel, and everyone feels—surprise!—younger than they actually happen to be. My hairdresser has this theory about what she calls "resting hair rate." It's similar to your resting heart rate, except it means that no matter what you do to your hair, it will resolve itself into some general style that is its natural fallback position. I personally believe in a resting weight rate: that is, if you're exercising pretty regularly and eating like a normal person (as opposed to those times when your girlfriends have taken you to Vegas for the weekend and you're consuming ten thousand calories a day, most of them in bread, butter, alcohol, and chocolate), there is some weight that your body will naturally adopt.

So maybe there's a resting age rate—that is, the age you naturally feel. According to the Pew study, most adults over fifty feel at least ten years younger than their actual age. A third of those between sixty-five and seventy-four said they felt between one and two decades younger. On his seventieth birthday, Ringo Starr, still drumming, told an interviewer, "As far as I'm concerned, in my head I'm twenty-four." If you woke me from a sound sleep and shouted, "How old are you?" I suspect I'd mutter, "Forty-one."

It's interesting for me to consider that that's my resting age rate, and then to compare that moment in my life to this one. My life was fine at forty-one. I had published a novel, was writing a newspaper column, had three children in all-day school for the first time. (Every mother will understand that that last clause should come first in the sentence.) I had just started to work out for the first time in my life, which turned out to be good, and I occasionally found myself squinting at my needlepoint or my book, which turned out to be not so good. (The actor Kevin Bacon says the good news is that the eyes and the face go at the same time, so you can't see how you look.) I had most of the friends I have today and the same husband. My life was a bit crazy, it's true: sometimes I had to edit a column while the kids were having dinner, which meant there were too many slapdash meals and run-on sentences. Sometimes I had to interrupt dinner to take calls. I remember the day our son Christopher came downstairs and said, "Some man just called on your office phone, but I told him you couldn't talk because you were making dinner." That man was Jesse Jackson. Isn't working at home great?

Nearly two decades later, I still work at home, but the children no longer live here, although their rooms are preserved as shrines, complete with old posters and artwork and high school course notes crammed in the desk drawers. I've published a number of novels, had another column but gave it up, have added a few friends despite my insistence that I don't have room in my life for more friends. If you woke me up from a sound sleep and shouted, "How's sixty looking?" I would murmur, "Good. Really good." Better, in many ways, than forty-one.

The natural world, and the modern one, tell us a different story, a story about women who are past it because they are no longer fecund, no longer fertile, no longer alluring to men in the way they were when they were twenty-two. My friend Marc told me that his beehives were failing because he'd gotten too attached to the queen, who was past her prime: that is, she was four. In *The Hive and the Honey Bee,* a kind of bible of beekeeping he lent me, it couldn't be clearer: "Aging queens are superseded, swarm queens are replaced with young ones." (Just to be clear, queens are replaced by killing them. Beekeeping is a little like presiding over the court of Henry VIII, only with honey.) In Hollywood they are sometimes similarly blunt. As the actress Lillian Gish once said, "You know, when I first went into the movies, Lionel Barrymore played my grandfather. Later he played my father, and finally he played my husband. If he had lived, I'm sure I would have played his mother. That's the way it is in Hollywood. The men get younger and the women get older."

But sometimes I think of that wonderful novel for young readers *Tuck Everlasting,* the story of a family whose members have drunk the waters of a stream that keep them forever frozen in time, and their insistence that immortality is a pestilence, that it interferes with the natural cycles of life, aging, and death. Kids who read the book always wind up arguing about whether they would take a drink despite the warnings of the Tuck family, and usually the younger they are, the more enamored they are of the notion of being young forever. But older children begin to understand the obvious peril: your friends, your parents, your siblings, your pets, will age and die and you will be left behind. In some inchoate way they begin to understand what their parents know and their grandparents understand deep down: that there is this rhythm to things, and that it is based in part on the young becoming older and giving way to the new young.

Most of us don't have tornadoes in our lives. Our disasters are manageable and predictable, the losses systematic and expected. The car conks out, a younger man is promoted in our stead, our incomes shrink, the heart goes haywire. Our grandparents die, then our mothers and fathers, then some of our friends. People manage to rebound from great devastation; we read about them every day, the parents who survive the death of a child (though we know we couldn't), the workers who lose lifelong jobs (a turn of affairs we're certain we wouldn't survive), the patients whose bodies are racked by terrible disease (which we wouldn't want to live with). And then sometimes we become one of those people and are amazed, not by our own strength but by that indomitable ability to slog through adversity, which looks like strength from the outside and just feels like every day when it's happening to you.

The older we get, the better we get at this. The older we get, the better we get at being ourselves. We're not busy being born, but busy being born again. My knee makes this noise like Rice Krispies when I do squats and lunges, and my dermatologist likes to joke that she has to clear her schedule when she checks my skin for age spots. But as my friend Robin Morgan, the writer and activist, said as she was approaching seventy, "Parts of me I never even knew I had sometimes ache—but parts of me I never knew I had in my brain *sing*."

So much of our knee-jerk negative response to aging is a societal construct. It's yet another version of the conflict that shapes, sometimes deforms, our lives, the conflict between what we really want and what we're told we ought to desire. We are supposed to think that young is better. But we know deep inside, in the ways that count, that better is now. On the day my friend Lesley's first grandchild was born, she sent out a message that ended, "You're never too old to have the best day of your life."

I opened the screen door tentatively after the tornado was done, took the dogs, and went outside to relearn my immediate world. There were trees and branches everywhere and a wicker rocker from the front porch flung into the back field and beneath it two squirrels, unmarked as though they'd died as we all say we want to die, lapsed into a good night's sleep that never ends. And I thought, How in the world will we ever come back from this? How in the world will this place ever look the same? And a year went by, and then two, and it doesn't look the same, any more than I do. In two places on the banks of the pond, I found large pointed rocks slammed several inches into the dirt, rocks the wind turned into missiles, or weapons. And for a moment I considered that if the dogs and I had been walking around the pond as we often do, one of those rocks could have hurtled toward me and done the kind of damage my daughter so feared.

But, for whatever reason, that didn't happen. It's not because there's any grand plan to the universe, it's just that life is various, millions of moving parts, dogs, stones, high winds, sandwiches, squirrels, tornadoes. There was a time when I behaved as though I was the center of that universe. It was a good time, when I was young, and arrogant, and foolish, and eager, and terribly insecure and horribly insensible to others and not beholden to anyone else, without responsibility for houses or children or dogs or the cleanup after a disaster. I just like this time better.

Push

My friends and I gave birth to our children at the dawn of an unfortunate era of übermomism unknown to past generations, or, as my mother-in-law once said, "If no one was bleeding, things were fine." This was more or less the standard of my own childhood, too, which was careless and carefree. If you had asked my mother at any given time where I was, she would likely have paused from spooning Gerber's peas into a baby's mouth and replied, "She's around here somewhere." In other words, by modern standards of mothering, that dictate that she ought to have known precisely where I was, perhaps because I was taking mini-Mandarin or having a playdate, my mother was a bust. (She also predated the term "playdate.") There's one problem with that conclusion. It's dead wrong. My mother was great at what she did; most of what I've brought to the table of motherhood she set out first. She didn't help us build with our Erector sets, didn't haul us to piano lessons. She couldn't even drive. But where she was always felt like a safe place.

I knew, without really thinking, that if I had kids I was going to get out of bed each day (or often, it turned out, in the middle of the night) and try to be as much like my own mother as possible. Kind and loving and always available with pepper-onion-and-egg sandwiches with melted mozzarella cheese. Who could ask for more?

The idea that kind and loving is enough is a tough sell in our current culture, and not simply because if one of my kids had wandered from home there would have been a caseworker and a cop at the door. We live in a perfection society now, and nowhere has that become more powerful—and more pernicious—than in the phenomenon of manic motherhood. What the child-care guru D. W. Winnicott once called "the ordinary devoted mother" is no longer enough. Instead there is the over-scheduled mom who bounces from soccer field to school fair to music lessons until she falls into bed at the end of the day, exhausted, her life somewhere between the Stations of the Cross and a decathlon.

A perfect storm of trends and events contributed to this. One was the teeter-totter scientific argument of nature versus nurture. When my mother was raising kids, there was a sub-rosa assumption that they were what they were. The smart one. The sweet one. Even the bad one. There was only so much a mother could do to mold the clay she'd been given. But as I became a mother myself, all that was changing. Little minds, we learned from researchers, were infinitely malleable, even before birth. Don't get tense: tense moms make tense infants. (That news'll make you tense!) I remember lying on the mat in a pre-natal exercise class, working on what was left of my stomach muscles, listening to the instructor repeating, "Now hug your baby." If I had weak abs, did that mean my baby went unhugged?

Keeping up with the Joneses turned into keeping up with the Joneses' kids. Whose mothers, by the way, all lied. I now refuse to believe in nine-month-olds who speak in full sentences. But I was more credulous then, and more vulnerable, when I had a nine-month-old myself. Never mind that twenty-month-old who wasn't ambulatory. If I unearthed the purse I carried then, which was huge, since it had to hold the diapers and the Wet Wipes and the Peas-and-Carrots food mill, because, ambulatory or not, the boy had to have fresh-milled food, I know I would find inside the scrawled names of pediatric neurologists given to me by several helpful women on the playground, where my son just sat and smiled and stared at his own hands while the other kids whirled around him.

How better to circumvent the power of the new women of our generation than with all this nonsense that made it seem that every moment was a teachable moment—and every teachable moment missed a measure of a lousy mom. We were part of the first generation of women who took it for granted that we would work not only throughout our lifetimes but throughout our children's childhoods as well. In 1976, Dr. Spock revised his bible of child care to say that this was fine, but he didn't explain how it would be possible, and there was a slapdash approach to melding our disparate roles. My first sitter was the erstwhile manager of a cult punk band. She was a good sitter, too.

But quicker than you could say nanny cam, books appeared, seminars were held, and modern motherhood was codified as a profession. Professionalized for women who didn't work outside the home: if they were giving up such supposedly great opportunities, then the tending of kids needed to be made into an all-encompassing job. Professionalized for women who had paying jobs out in the world: to show that their work was not bad for their kids, they just had to take childrearing as seriously as they did dealmaking.

It turned out that this was not such a good thing. It wasn't only that baking for the bake sale, meeting with the teachers, calling the other mothers about the sleepover, and scoping out the summer camp made women of all sorts crazy, turning stress from an occasional noun into an omnipresent verb and adverb. A lot of this oversight was not particularly good for kids, either. If your mother has been micromanaging your homework since you were six, it's hard to feel any pride of ownership when you do well. You can't learn from mistakes and disappointments if your childhood is engineered so there aren't any.

And much of this didn't end with childhood anyhow. What came to be called helicopter parenting extended into adolescence, so that colleges looked at some admissions essays with skepticism, wondering how much they'd been massaged into shape by anxious parents, or by professionals the anxious parents hired. College deans reported that it was commonplace to hear directly from parents unhappy with a grade or a roommate assignment; on moving-in day a dean at our daughter's college handed out cards that read "How are *you* going to deal with that problem?" and suggested that we read the sentence, exactly as written, when we got telephone calls with complaints from our kids.

I mark my years of parenting by the people who stepped in and forced me to abandon my inclination to meddle, micromanage, and coddle, beginning with my children's father, who sat me down and told me in year two that I was going to create a little monster if I continued to act as though "no" and "I don't love you" were synonymous. Also on my list is the high school college counselor who told the junior class parents, to the sound of strangled gasping, that they were forbidden to go on college visits with their sons. I thought of him again when I read a newspaper story about boomer parents who were actually accompanying their children—who by then were not children but adults—to job interviews.

I processed this remarkable and deeply troubling phenomenon in two ways. As someone who once did hiring, I would have rejected immediately and out of hand any young person whose mother or father was waiting for them in reception. But as someone who had to keep herself from sneaking into her kids' rooms to read their college essays and to do some judicious editing—oh, come on, they'll never notice that unfamiliar metaphor in the middle of their own prose—I understood the impulse. I just vowed not to give in to it. How could they be excited about their jobs, their opinions, their lives, if they felt that they were secondhand, jerry-built, not truly their own, if they weren't discovering the world anew?

Oh, sure, there's something a tiny bit wearing about that, about their idealism, their illusions, the intense vagaries of sensation and emotion. I have to remind myself of the time when I was young and seeing a man who was nearly twenty years my senior. He was a wonderful person in almost every way, except that everything I wanted to do, he'd already done. Douglas Sirk movies, Positano, truffles, Italian tailoring: he knew, and I was learning, and it made for an unbreachable disconnect. Each time I've been tempted to tell one of the kids they'll get over it, whatever it is—love affair, crippled friendship, failure at school—I would remember this. I couldn't afford to be world-weary. One study found that nearly all of those in their twenties, asked if they agree with the statement "I am very sure that someday I will get to where I want to be in life," say yes. That should be cause for celebration, not pursed lips and a cynical *ha!* They will get to that place soon enough.

Besides, what kind of fool would I be to miss the opportunity to feel the sharp elbows of sensation again, to reexperience life vicariously, armed with the long view? Because naturally at some level this is all about us. Our relationships with our kids epitomize that old joke: Enough about me. What about you? What do you think about me? It places each of us squarely in the center of one of the great tugs-of-war of human existence, between connection and independence.

The thirst for novelty versus the hunger for security explains why some marriages blow up and others endure, why some people have spectacular careers and others just ricochet from passing interest to passing interest. There's the yen to contract, to draw in and have and do less, and the spur to spread out, to travel and explore. There's the tension between emotion and thought, between even temper and high anxiety. When we're young, many of us, there's a constant pendulum moving between the two, too high one way, too high another. But there comes that moment when we settle down, or settle in, or just settle.

There comes that moment when we give our children custody of their own selves or blight their lives forever, when we understand that being a parent is not transactional, that we do not get what we give. It is the ultimate pay-it-forward endeavor: we are good parents not so they will be loving enough to stay with us but so they will be strong enough to leave us. Modern mythology has it that this happens suddenly, overnight, with something called the empty nest. But that wasn't the case in this household. There are three of them, so when one, even two went to college there was still one left at home. Ah, how foolish she was: after years of having her brothers lord it over her, smack her down, infantilize her, she thought being the only child would be fantastic, when it turned out to be mainly lonely. "And the two of you are so focused on me!" she told her father and me more than once. Once she went off, her brothers began to circle back, until finally all three wound up in New York City, available for emergency dogsitting and Sunday evening pizza and TV sporting events. Occasionally I come home and find a cereal bowl in the sink with a slick of milk in the bottom, and I know I should think, Why can't they wash their own dishes; they're grown now, what am I, the maid? Our children are occasional visitors with all the rights and privileges of full-time residents, which is an uncomfortable combination. But still I smile, and put the bowl in the dishwasher. The nest has been visited.

But it is still just a visit. My friend Gail, who has always provided dispatches from the foreseeable future because her children are just a little older than ours—and who once provided a gently used crib and changing table, too—warned me that it was really after graduation that the feeling of being downsized hit with full force. Work schedules that undermine family holiday celebrations, significant others who want to lay claim to Thanksgiving. A Venn diagram in which their circles overlap ours less and less. I built my entire existence around our children, wrote only during school hours, didn't write at all when there was a school vacation or an ear infection. In the same way that I go dark around the anniversary of my mother's death without really knowing at first what's happening, so at around three some days when I'm working at home, I feel a spasm of loneliness, like a spiritual charley horse. No one is waiting for me to pick them up at school. My poor husband eats the same dish, reheated in Corning glass, for weeks, because I am incapable of making cassoulet or sauce Bolognese for two. No, actually, I'm not incapable. I'm unwilling. Someone may drop by, someone I once nursed, dressed, read to, yelled at, cooked for every day. When they were young, there was a schedule, a shape to things. How many for dinner—that is the essential question.

Of course it's not. The essential questions are much more cosmic, more critical, more terrifying. Who will they marry? What will they do with their professional lives? Will they have children, and will those children thrive? There were once bright lines to mothering, when they were little. You cannot cross the street without holding my hand. You cannot have a cookie until after dinner. Even later on, as they grew, there were curfews and rules. When my children came home at night during the teenage years, I would wait up, hug them close, and inhale deeply, sniffing for the smell of beer or pot. None of them missed the narc beneath the embrace. Our relationship was shaped by that constant duality, too, by love and fear. For instance: let's say you have a teenage son who arrives home from camp and tosses his duffel to the bottom of the basement stairs so that it comes to rest, beseeching, against the maw of the washing machine. The clothes within will be divided into three groups: those that require hot water, those that require hot water and full-strength bleach, and those that need to be chucked. The duffel is up-ended onto the basement floor, and amid the filthy socks and mildewed shorts, bright as bits of foil-wrapped candy, lie a dozen condoms. Time stops, and the mother brain divides into two parts:

- *He got the message about safe sex.*
- *He's having sex.*

Once our children have moved into adulthood, the messages are more poignant, more complex, and, if we're smart, more often unspoken unless solicited. Instead of crossing the street, they are navigating a work world where we cannot follow. The beer in the fist is sanctioned by law and by custom. And in our sinking hearts we begin to realize that while they know about safe sex, they are only beginning to understand that there is no such thing as safe love. It is one thing to tell a ten-year-old she cannot watch an R-rated movie; it is another to watch her, at age thirty, preparing to marry a man you are convinced will not make her happy. I remember the profound, almost physical sense of relief I felt when I understood that our sons and daughter did not have colic, were not autistic, showed no signs of adolescent mental illness. Done, I thought, licking my finger and crossing those things off the blackboard in my mind. When did I realize that there was something more terrifying, the possibility that any of them might have to struggle with a child with those problems, that heartrending moment when you face not your own difficult challenges but those that might come to the people you love most? Was it that evening, lying in bed and talking about my mother's cancer and genetics, when out of the dark my husband's voice asked, "So Maria's at risk?" The fact that that question came as a complete shock to me, so well versed in medicine, so thoughtful about heredity, must be a reflection of the denial that covers us, like a hood, when bad things might happen to our kids. Little children, little problems; big children, big problems. Why do people share that dictum? It can't be reassuring to anyone.

Nor is it soothing to let them loose to make their own decisions and mistakes. But it is the entire point of the exercise, shifting the balance, giving them a little more rope each year. I remember when he was in fifth grade and Quin, our eldest, came to me to complain that he had had the same bedtime his entire life. I was so busy that I'd forgotten to let him stay up until 9:00 P.M., which felt like something of an epic fail. On the other hand, we knew parents who let their children dictate their own bedtimes so they could develop a sense of mastery and control. Which, by the way, is something no nine-year-old actually needs.

It's all in the calibrations over the long haul. When we think of longer life expectancy, we may envision ten years added to our existence later on. But it may also be that we've added time to adolescence, which now stretches past the teen years and into the twenties. So much has been written about how the young people of America seem to stay young longer now, well past the time when their grandparents owned houses and had families, and some of that surely has to do with a life expectancy that makes the forced march into adulthood slightly more leisurely. But it's also true that their grandparents never had a mother calling the teacher to complain about a bad grade. And they certainly didn't have parents who would call the college dean; my father's sole connection with my higher education was when he dropped me off freshman year, and when he came back for commencement. I would have felt so diminished if he had ever called one of my professors, but luckily the idea would never have occurred to him.

I liked to congratulate myself on my restraint when I would hear stories about parents who micromanaged their sons' and daughters' college courses or job decisions, but the truth is, part of this was garden-variety sloth. I didn't want to work that hard. I passed on the weekend roundelay of kiddy-league sports when they were younger so our three could hang out with one another. I told people I hoped it would cement a bond among them, and it did. But I really wanted to be reading rather than standing on the sidelines pretending my kids were soccer prodigies. Maybe I had three children in the first place so I wouldn't ever have to play board games. In my religion, martyrs die.

Quin wrested custody of his life away from me at a fairly early age, perhaps inspired by a bout, shame-making in memory, in which I tried to persuade him to rewrite a perfectly good fourth-grade paper to turn it into an eighth-grade paper. I'd been addled by the class art projects, some of which looked like the work of a crack graphic design team—and were. He was wiser than I was; I didn't set eyes on his college essay until he'd mailed his applications, and I knew immediately that it was going to either instantly disqualify him or be his ticket in. It was the latter, which was a good thing for his brother and sister, since the niggling suspicion that I would have tried to persuade him to homogenize his essay, perhaps to ill effect, led me to be hands-off with them. So, once again, do the younger ones benefit from our experiments on the eldest, who got me used to myself. When Maria had her wisdom teeth removed, I doled out the heavy-duty opiates; when Quin had his done, I didn't even fill the prescription. "I'm so sorry about the Vicodin, honey," I said as he sat with his sister. "It's okay, Mom," he replied evenly. "I only had two out at a time."

I asked him once about his memories of my mothering, and yes, I know I was taking a big chance there, but in his dealings with me he has grown to be almost as kind and gentle as he is with his grandparents. "You sorta freaked out during the college application process," he noted accurately. But then he wrote, "What I remember most: having a good time."

There's the problem with turning motherhood into martyrdom. There's no way to do it and have a good time. The most incandescent memories of my childhood are of making my mother laugh. My kids do the same for me. Nobody has ever managed to crack me up the way Quin, Chris, and Maria Krovatin have, except maybe their father.

Sometimes on the way to the circus, or the car, or around the pond, the three kids walk side by side, their heads bent together, their words a kind of pigeon murmur, alto and undecipherable, and Gerry and I will exchange a half smile that means, my God, how did this happen? The alchemy of parenthood is so mysterious. It can't be true that we were somehow responsible for creating these three unique and remarkable human beings. We didn't know enough, do enough. There were endless diaper changes, baths, books, Band-Aids, doctor visits, parent-teacher conferences, plays and athletic events and family dinners, so much scut work. It's as though we were working long repetitive shifts on an assembly line, and in the end we had the Sistine Chapel.

I had no clue about how they would change everything. That sounds preposterous, since both my husband and I are the eldest in largish families and both of us had childhoods punctuated by pregnancies, the weeklong disappearance of our mothers, and the arrival of yet another lozenge of a receiving blanket with a red face and a querulous cry. But being supplanted by babies was quite different from being in thrall to them. Giving birth to a baby is one thing; it's another to realize you've given birth to a man. I don't mean changing a diaper and getting sprayed in the sternum; I mean walking someone to kindergarten and helping him put on his fake beard for the Purim play, and then one day turning around to discover that he has a real beard, and an Adam's apple, and a bass voice, and boxer shorts. I am the mother now of two grown men, who are bigger than I am and in many ways smarter, who know how to tie a tie and throw a football, neither of which I have ever mastered.

And I am the mother of a woman, too. She started out very picky about her party dresses, and she liked to pretend she was the Little Mermaid, standing at the top of the stairs and warbling, "I'm coming, Prince Erik!" And then suddenly she was inveighing against sexism and giving her friends relationship advice. You look at her and understand how it's not only possible but also desirable to be utterly female and terribly confident. You realize that instead of your being her role model, the tables have turned.

It was an education, raising these children, but mainly for me, not so much for them. There was the sense of competence that motherhood conferred, that sense that if we could handle Halloween or the first day of school or a rainy week in midsummer, we would be able to handle anything. By the time I had all three I was no longer doing hiring, but had I been I suspect I would have mainly hired mothers returning to the work world because I would have known they could handle several things at once and still manage to peel out of the office at a reasonable hour.

Having and raising my children made me better than myself, but they did something else as well: they helped me learn to grow older. Sometimes I think about how, on my birthdays, the first words out of my father's mouth are always, "Wow, I must be getting really old!" For a long time I thought this was because my father has a way of putting himself at the center of any event—the baby at every christening, the bride at every wedding, the corpse at every funeral, as someone once said of Teddy

Roosevelt—but like many things my father has told me, it resonates now as it couldn't when I was younger. My place in the span of life is what my kids have shown me, too. Just as, when they were small and we were in charge of every aspect of their lives, we couldn't help but feel like responsible adults (or, on occasion, faux responsible adults), so when I see my grown children, I can't deny my own progression. I am part of an unbroken wave, but I am no longer its leading edge. Sometimes I look at photographs of all of us together and for an instant my mind registers an error, of angle, of perspective. Who is that very short woman at the center of the scrum? Everyone towers over me. "Little Mommy," Christopher says occasionally, fondly.

Any equanimity I bring to this process of growing older, of getting slower, of ceding the center to others, I've gotten from them. They forced me to relearn the catechism of self: instead of focusing all the time on how they ought to behave, who they ought to be, I tried to focus on who they really were. In the process I finally got a handle on who I really was. In coming to understand that Quin's unwavering certainty and responsibility were a thin veneer over deep emotion and constant self-examination, I came to understand and even appreciate the same about myself. In accepting Christopher's overweening individuality and lack of conformity, I dared to take my own steps in that direction. And Maria's audacity and fearlessness made me push myself away from the beckoning quicksand of the compliant girl who had somehow survived within me despite my years of exorcisms. A long time ago, over the space of five years, a balding doctor with the benevolent look of a kindly goat peered up at me and said, "Push!" Little did I understand that that was what I would have to do from then on—push to do right for their sake, push to be better because of their example. The older I get, the more I want to be like them.

Expectations

We've lived through a time of incredible challenge, many of us, in which we've been trying to be both our mother and our father simultaneously. But I feel as though it's been the very best time to live, that those of us of a certain age got it all, like a time-lapse photograph, branch to bud to blossom in a single generation.

We started with a world of virtually no options, then moved on to a time in which every bit of progress seemed like a battle, in which valedictorians at good colleges who happened to be female were still assumed to be seeking work they would pursue only until they got engaged, or got pregnant. And then suddenly we could be anywhere, do anything, except for pope and president, and no woman really wants that first job anyway, and we will sooner or later get the second. It's been like the Industrial Revolution without sweatshops, or the American Revolution without blood. Victory was ours, but not without some suffering. "Oh, you poor girls, with all your choices," an older woman once said to me during an interview. And I knew exactly what she meant. There have been times when it required two or three people to be a reasonably competent version of me. But I'm not complaining.

It's hard to begin to explain to our children and their friends how radically different the expectations have become in the years between my birth and their own. That's it, really: the expectations. The idea of who we are and what we can do. My mother knew she was never going to college; the expectation was that she would marry and have children and that therefore higher education would be wasted. My father's attitude toward me was the polar opposite. The most shocking announcement I ever made to him was that I was pregnant. "What about your job?" he said. He believed in a world that was either-or, in which I could be a success at work or as a mother but not both, and certainly not at the same time.

I understood his reaction. I'd been a child in an either-or world, in which the career choices I faced were to be either a mother or a nun. As a child, I saw no women in positions of real power and authority. Perhaps as important, I saw no women who worked for pay. The money women had was given to them by men. The position they held was given to them by men. And believe me, for a girl who was outspoken, intelligent, insurrectionary, and always faintly pissed off, that was a powerful goad to think the world needed changing.

And change it did. The greatest social tsunami of my lifetime, the women's movement, was part fearsome political force, part personal support group. It was hated and feared, and it changed the world completely, so that sometimes I want to send its leaders a note that says, "Thank you for my life." With all the technological changes of the last half century, it's the women's movement that has provided the greatest change in the way we live now. My daughter once asked me if a man could be secretary of state, a job I grew up believing would only be held by men. But during Maria's youth the position had been occupied by Madeleine Albright, Condoleezza Rice, and Hillary Clinton. Colin Powell must have seemed like a fluke.

That's progress, but it's also an interesting problem. The social movement that changed my life has been hugely successful, but it's not over. It only seems that way. Obviously it's easier to sell the necessity of the labor union movement when young women caught in a fire in the Triangle Shirtwaist Factory die than when people on automobile assembly lines are making an hourly wage three or four times higher than the minimum. It's easier to argue against racial prejudice when drinking fountains are designated black and white and a young black man who whistles at a white woman can be murdered with impunity than it is when the question is how many black kids are going to get into Harvard and whether the black son of a doctor is given a leg up over the white son of a cop.

It's far easier to argue for the systematic devaluing of women if women are denied the right to own property, to take the bar exam, and to say no to their husbands than it is when women are merely finding it hard to get elected president. There are so many glasses half full: female cops and firefighters, female Supreme Court justices and senators. But for every one there is a glass half empty, too: the harassment female law-enforcement officers still face, the women soldiers who fear rape from their fellows as well as the enemy, the justices who still have to calibrate their fashion choices for the confirmation hearings, the senators who find it harder to raise money than even their dopiest male colleagues. It's not just that some jerks yelled, "Iron my shirts!" at Hillary Clinton when she was running for president, or that someone asked the Republican candidate, John McCain, "How are we going to beat the bitch?" It's that no one acted as though either of those things was that big a deal.

When prejudice, bigotry, and injustice are entrenched, egregious, and sanctioned, we're looking at big-muscle-group remedies—the lawsuit, the amendments, the marches. But we're now more often in the small-muscle-group area, the business of personal behavior and attitudes. After Sandra Day O'Connor was chosen to be the first woman on the United States Supreme Court in 1981, one of the letters she received read, "Back to your kitchen and home female! This is a job for a man and only he can make the tough decisions. Take care of your grandchildren and husband." The truth is that that sort of nonsense made the early movement for women's equality simpler. Fighting that kind of flagrant bigotry requires less finesse than sidling around tokenism or dealing with entrenched custom. Young women today encounter the subtle sexism of far-enough rather than the raw stuff of no-way. At the sort of firms from which the job-seeking O'Connor was summarily turned away after her graduation from Stanford Law at mid-century, there are now plenty of female lawyers. But most power is still concentrated in white men, white men who hire those who remind them of themselves when young.

The next generation of women may bust past that as they move into the second stage of this revolution, in part because they're growing up with, befriending, and marrying young men who have been raised in this new world by mothers who have been living its precepts. Raising feminist boys was the great challenge of my life, and it wasn't easy for them; it wasn't about dolls instead of trucks—both of mine preferred Lego blocks— but about getting them to refuse the easy assumption of privilege and the unconscious assumption of superiority, which, let's face it, is challenging for anyone. But, as our son Chris remarked once, chicks dig it. My sons like and respect women, which women, unsurprisingly, find attractive. My daughter likes and respects herself, which means at some seminal (ovular) level, my work here at home is done.

But our work in the world is not. I'm struck by the plateaus inherent in great change, especially at the most basic level. All the times I've been asked on college campuses about balancing work and family, I've never been asked the question by a young man. Young women, even with their own mothers' successes, wonder how they will manage job and kids; young men still figure they'll manage it by marrying.

Even though we no longer have to rush out of the office with some lame excuse about a family emergency when what actually happened is that our fifth-grader threw up onto his math book, we're still feeling that double standard for women. And we're feeling it at both ends of the family life continuum. Recently I got an email from a friend that was representative of an entire shift in the way we live now: "In Boston getting our daughter settled in her apartment then on to Vermont to move my mother into assisted living."

We are the first generation of women who are intimately involved in the lives of our children and in the lives of our parents while trying to hold down jobs outside the home at the same time. Someone even came up with a name for this: the sandwich generation. It is yet another way in which the actuarial charts make us distinct: while a hundred years ago fewer than 7 percent of those in their sixties had a living parent, today that number is almost 50 percent. At the same time, many more children over the age of eighteen are still living at home. The irony is rich—the women's movement taught us we could be more than caregivers, and now we're caregivers to more people than ever before. When it was first coined, the phrase "having it all" designated the doctor who went from the office to the soccer field to watch her kids play, then went home to a dinner cooked by her husband the architect. Now it more often means the doctor who is moving her mother into an assisted-living facility, monitoring the meds of her husband's parents who are still trying to get by in their own home, and waking in the middle of the night as her college graduate stomps up the stairs, partying off the strain of not being able to find a job, or not being able to find one that pays enough to rent an apartment.

We're working this out on the fly, with the help of other women, just as we did with the balancing of work and family, having the baby and keeping the job. Today the same women who called to ask one another how they were handling reading-readiness, early puberty, and SAT prep classes find themselves swapping advice about bone scans, nutritional supplements, and nursing homes. "You should call her," I heard one woman say of a mutual friend at lunch. "She knows everything about Alzheimer's."

The changes in the lives of women over the last half century and the extension of life expectancy have both coincided with a great migration. Extended families are scattered, easy access to aunts and uncles a thing of the past. My family didn't care for my kids while I worked; my paid family of sitters did. What the women's movement has often meant is the hiring of other women to do some of the work for us, from housekeepers to home health aides. Here was what passed for a retirement community during my childhood: after his wife died, my grandfather Pantano lived in a bedroom in a house with my aunt Mary and uncle Angelo, my cousins Maurice and Mary Jane. He tended tomato plants in the backyard wearing a white dress shirt, his iron-gray hair slicked straight back with some fragrant oil. It never occurred to me to ask if all involved liked this arrangement. It was how things worked. It was a smallish house, where they all lived. Today we have much bigger houses, but there is no room for grandparents to live there. Nor, in many cases, would they want to.

I don't remember hearing the phrase "assisted living" until I was well into adulthood. Sun City in Arizona, the first retirement community for "active seniors," is slightly younger than I am. Places like it now fill the landscape of the exurbs, planned communities to which those under fifty-five are cordially disinvited, where overnight visits from grandchildren are curtailed

in duration of stay. Americans are people who prize independence and autonomy. But for the aged, the infirm, and the enfeebled, that prize is often out of reach. Taking up the slack for
them is no longer a mission, it is a business. "Huge growth in the
nursing-home sector," one businessman said to me at dinner one
night, and I shivered.

All great social movements exact a price from someone, for
someone. We've created a new world that is still figuring itself
out, and one of the greatest conundrums is how women who
taught their daughters, by their example and their words, to be
strong and independent, to take control of their own future and
to take care of themselves, will navigate the dependency of old
age. My internist, who has many older patients, says she frequently encounters those who have persuaded their middle-
aged children that they are fine, that they need no help, that they
are perfectly content living independently. "Except," my doctor
adds, "it doesn't happen to be true." Some of these women, she
says, wind up moving in with one another for company and
support. That sounds about right to me. My plan is that a group
of us will move together into our house in the country, with a
crackerjack cook and a couple of aides. We'll repeat the same
stories, trash the same absent friends, secure in the knowledge
that none of us will notice the repetitions. Our children will call,
male and female alike, working, busy, with too much to do, and
we'll say, "Fine, dear. Nice to hear from you. Have to go."

Or maybe it won't be like that at all. Maybe we'll yearn for
the old days when one of the daughters-in-law would have been
guilted into giving us the guest bedroom, when we would tut-
tut about how much time she spent lunching with her friends
when she could be home cooking for her husband, who of course
would be incapable of cooking for himself. That all sounds so
antique, doesn't it? Despite the trade-offs, things seem fairer
now, even though the changes in women's lives have caused so

much upheaval. As my father once said to me feelingly, "Can you imagine what it would have been like if you had been born fifty years earlier? Your life would have been miserable."

Perhaps this will all work itself out for the next generation of young women. I hear a complaint all the time about them: They don't get it. They don't understand how hard we've worked to get here. They don't understand how bad things were. They don't understand that you used to have to keep your mouth shut if your boss made a grab at you, or that no matter how smart you were or where you'd gone to college the first question anyone asked at a job interview was, "Can you type?"

But how in the world do we expect them to feel the utterly changed tenor of the times any more than I can truly feel what it was like for my grandparents to raise a houseful of children during the Depression? Of course I know the history, and at home I've heard the stories. But personal experience is the trump card.

Progress is always relative. Sometimes it's not even real. I once heard Claudia Kennedy, at the time the only three-star female general in the Army, talk about the question of critical mass, of how many members of any group you need inside the tent before you can speak up, speak out, make change, raise hell. But maybe there's a critical mass at which it seems as though things are dandy when dandy is still a way off. Is it fourteen women in the Senate? Is it three women on the Supreme Court? It's amazing how few women are required on a corporate board to satisfy the suits that they've done the woman thing. Actually, it's not just corporations. For years I was a journalism show pony, trotted out to prove a point, at some conference, on some panel: John, Joe, James, and me, there to send a message that women were well represented, in newspapers, in opinion writing, and in the public discourse of the country. None of which was true.

A few years ago there was a report from the White House

Project that showed there was a lid on big jobs for women, a lid set at roughly 20 percent. Half the population and, on average, only 20 percent of the country's leaders, in business, in journalism, in law, in politics. In many cases women's participation had been stuck at that level for years while other countries moved ahead. The United States had dropped down the world's ladder of female political representation to a position behind countries like Iraq and North Korea. At big law firms one study showed that women were a measly 12 percent of partners in 1993. Fifteen years later, that number was up to 18 percent. Hearts and minds may have been won, but bodies in the boardroom hadn't followed.

When you talk about that, someone always says that women opt out, for home and family or because they don't want the punishing hours that partnership or high position demands. People have been saying that my whole life long, that women don't run things because deep down inside they don't want to. Instead of that excuse, I always wonder why no one wonders why the standard-issue top job is considered so heinous that a whole class of people, people who often manage to deal with explosive diarrhea and projectile vomiting—occasionally at the same time—would pass on it. And maybe it's the job that's passed on them, not the other way around. I once had a boss who would praise any woman he considered especially promising by saying that someday she could be managing editor. He thought that was a big deal: in those days no woman had come close to a job that big. The only problem was that managing editor was the number two spot, and it was hard to believe that anyone would tell some guy that he was such a star that he might rocket to the second spot. One crazy day I said that. My boss looked at me as though I'd lost my mind. Lack of gratitude, sense of entitlement—that's what he was thinking.

Besides, I'm not sure whether the young women of today will hit the glass ceiling hardest in the office or in the world.

They certainly won't know what it is like to watch as their fathers and husbands go out to vote for president and they have to stay home. They won't know what it is like to be denied entry to West Point or even to basic training.

Maybe they will hit the glass ceiling at home, when almost overnight the world implodes, when they are transformed from junior executives with the world on a microchip to homebound mothers with two kids under the age of three and oatmeal in their hair, hit it when they realize that they have wound up with two full-time jobs and their male counterparts have not because of unfinished business about the division of those jobs formerly designated women's work. Maybe they will hit the glass ceiling even later than that, when they realize that if their aged parents need help, the women of the family are still expected to provide it. My grandmother used to recite a little ditty: A son is a son till he takes a wife, but a daughter's a daughter the rest of her life. I always thought it had ominous undertones. When my father demanded that I quit college to care for my mother when she was ill, I occasionally made bitter comments about the tradition of Irish Catholic households sacrificing their daughters for the greater good. But it wasn't just my father, and it wasn't just the Irish, and it wasn't just then.

Maybe, in tandem with this new generation of young men, women will develop real partnerships, real divisions of labor, on this front and so many others. I wish the women of my generation had, but we didn't. In general we still wound up doing more, scheduling playdates as well as business meetings, listening to distraught colleagues at work and then listening to distraught kids at home. Of the work that needed to be done, women did much, much more than their fair share, either the woman of the house or the women they hired to be their surrogates there.

I hope this changes for my children. I'm happy they were

spared the decades of lousy contraception and forced pregnancies, spared the quotas at professional schools and the punitive laws that held, for instance, that a rape could only be prosecuted if a third party witnessed the attack (preferably, I assume, a police officer or a priest). I'm happy they live in a world in which it is regularly acknowledged that a man who hits his wife is a bully and a weakling, and a man who takes care of his own children is not babysitting, and a man who changes diapers is not entitled to be treated as though he's just invented fire. So much seems normative for them: the stay-at-home dad down the street, the woman presidential candidate, the mother who does not defer, the father who does not insist on the last word. It's not that all the problems of gender disparity have been solved—far from it. There are different problems now, issues of nuance and unspoken assumption instead of the blunt club of bigotry and supremacy. There's still plenty to be done.

But still, it is hard to explain to them how different the expectations have become, how utterly transformed our lives have been over their course. When I came to *The New York Times* as a reporter in 1978, at age twenty-five, I thought I'd been hired because I was aces at my job. It took me a few months to figure out that a small group of courageous women had sued the paper and that the hiring of a bumper crop of female reporters and editors, what I thought of as the class of 1978, was the result.

Fast-forward to a June morning in 2011, when a woman named Jill Abramson became the first woman to run the paper. One of the women who had been a plaintiff in that suit wrote this comment: "Women of the NY Times who participated in historic 1978 sex discrimination class action suit—at last here is our highest reward."

Of course it wasn't exactly their reward. In the way of these things, the women who brought suit didn't prosper much. I did, and my fellow female reporters as well. We were hired, and promoted, and even considered suitable for the second spot on the masthead someday. And then, on one historic day, one of us was promoted to the top job. Perhaps the next generation will not even find that notable because it will have become so commonplace. Unremarkable equality, that's what they've grown up with. What a legacy we've left them, male and female alike.

PART IV

The Be-All and End-All

As I give thought to the matter, I find four causes for the apparent misery of old age; first, it withdraws us from active accomplishments; second, it renders the body less powerful; third, it deprives us of almost all forms of enjoyment; fourth, it stands not far from death.

—Cicero

One day I asked my friend Steve, who writes music, why "Taps" makes you feel the way it does. I figured there was some combination of notes that gives us that feeling of exaltation and sadness each time a trumpeter plays those few short bars. Steve said he thought it was mainly a matter of tempo and association: that music played slowly in a funeral setting inevitably created the emotions I described. To prove his point, he dum-dummed "Taps" in a much more sprightly fashion and it did sound different, more Sousa and less Elgar, more cheer and less mourning.

Perhaps that's the key to getting older, that how you feel about it has to do with context, the combination of past associations and current tempo.

I believe that there are essential mysteries, things written on the body that we sense and still cannot quite figure out or define. The future is one of them. It's not so much that it's unknowable as that it's unfeelable. It seems to be a country populated by vague characters who are Not Us. Thinking about it always reminds me of the scene in *A Christmas Carol* in which Scrooge is traveling in the future with the Ghost of Christmas Yet to Come and keeps looking around for himself. He suspects he doesn't see himself because he's changed so much; it turns out he doesn't see himself because he's in the churchyard, six feet under. "Are these the shadows of things that will be, or are they shadows of things that may be, only?" he asks the spirit.

Well, that is the question, isn't it? Is there a certain predestination to our lives from here on in, an existence that is inevitable because of all that has gone before? At what point is the clay set, the mural done and signed? Or does it all depend on whether we see our swan song as a dirge or a ditty?

At age sixty I find myself poised between the inevitable and the possible, the things I know and understand and the things I hope to learn and perhaps unravel. But it's still a bit of a mystery, the yet to come, with that greatest of all mysteries, mortality, at its very end.

In her beautiful memoir of life after sixty, *The Last Gift of Time,* Carolyn Heilbrun writes, so sensibly, "Since we do not wish to die, surely we must have wished to grow old." Aging, dying: both are a challenge to the human imagination. As the carapace of wrinkles and sag develops, we persist in seeing ourselves otherwise, so that when we peer into the mirror it is our own eyes we look into, the ones that have looked back at us since we were children. That child within each of us gives us hope that there will be more to learn, to discover, more to change and understand.

Faith

I waited a long time for a sister. Or at least it felt like a long time, which makes sense since I was a child and everything feels like it takes forever when you're seven or eight. What's the old motto? For the young the days go fast and the years go slow; for the old the days go slow and the years go fast. The years during which I had a brother, then another, then another, seemed to go very slowly. Then one morning in April my father came home from the hospital and announced that I had a sister. And for some utterly bizarre reason my parents had decided that I could name her.

My sister's name is Theresa Bernadette.

Many people reading that name would consider it either slightly strange or rather old-fashioned. But for Catholic girls of a certain era, it makes perfect sense. My sister is named for what any of us would consider the Big Two: Saint Thérèse of Lisieux, the French saint known as the Little Flower, a high-strung child who spent most of her youth trying to persuade clerical officials to let her follow her sister into a Carmelite monastery, and Saint

Bernadette of Lourdes, the peasant girl who had visions of a beautiful lady in a rock declension who the church eventually concluded was the Virgin Mary, turning Bernadette's hometown into a mecca for pilgrims seeking cures. There was even a Hollywood movie of her life, which for Catholic saints is comparatively rare. The beautiful Jennifer Jones played Bernadette.

For me, being Catholic is like being Irish or Italian or Caucasian, not a faith but an immutable identifying characteristic with which I was born and with which I will die. Many of the faithful would not consider this so; they would point to the fact that I no longer attend Mass every Sunday and never followed church directives on contraception. (If I had, I would be writing now about the challenges of raising twelve children.) But the Church is in the schools I attended, the women who taught me, the way I dressed and ate and spent my days as a child, the way I raised my own children and buried the older members of my extended family. It is woven into the fabric of my self, in both the warp and woof, so that it seems if you pulled its threads, all the rest would unravel. If a stranger were to stop me on the street and say, "The Lord be with you," I would reply automatically, just as I did for many years during Mass, "And also with you." Or perhaps "And with your spirit," which is what the response once was and then became again, or even *"Et cum spiritu tuo,"* the Latin of the Church of my childhood.

I am a long way from those traditionalists who chart the decline of modern Catholicism from the moment when its rituals were couched in a language its people could actually understand, but I sometimes think the modern translators lacked a sense of the poetry of prose. I still prefer to recall that Mary gave birth to Jesus and placed him in a manger because there was no room at the inn; the first time I heard the revamped version of the Gospel that instead spoke of "the place where travelers lodged," I cringed. It sounded as though the Holy Family got shut out of a cut-rate motel. No room at the inn. That's what happened.

The bedrock of my life as a reader and as a writer is in these stories from the New Testament, of an angel appearing to Mary and saying, "Fear not," of Jesus changing water into wine at a wedding. ("We'll save the best wine for last, like Cana," my husband said one night when friends came for dinner, and once again I was grateful that I married what seemed like the only Catholic boy at Columbia.) More important, the bedrock of my life as a citizen and a human being is contained in my faith as well. As I've said often, much to the consternation of friends of other faiths who have come to see Catholicism as narrow, conservative, and antediluvian, I am a liberal because I was raised Catholic. In a typically thoughtful and searching speech he gave at Notre Dame, former New York governor Mario Cuomo, the most intellectual of nonclerical Catholics, referred to practicing the work of Christ in our life, "practicing it especially where that love is most needed, among the poor and the weak and the dispossessed." That's the lesson I took away from the New Testament, the requirement that if you had two cloaks you should give one to the person who had none, that you should love your neighbor as yourself. It's a lesson that has never left me.

But what has disappeared, the older I've gotten, is the kind of belief that I once thought I would have forever. I began, as a child, by accepting that certain things were true, things that I would learn, as I grew older, were considered odd and even bizarre by others. The idea that the bread and wine at Communion had become the body and blood of Christ, the idea that Christ was the Son of God, the notion that Mary gave birth although she was a virgin. Of course, when we first learned this it was a more innocent time, when none of us knew what a virgin really was.

Naturally, when I was a teenager I was disdainful, of the

Church, of its traditions, even of its underlying messages. During four years of college I attended Mass only when I was at home and my parents insisted. Yet when I was living in lower Manhattan, alone, with no one to roust me on Sunday mornings (often with a hangover), I found myself occasionally at the church of St. Anthony of Padua on nearby Sullivan Street, just north of the salumeria that made fresh mozzarella, surrounded by women who could have been cousins of the Guarinis and Pantanos, who were my maternal relations.

It's commonplace for parents to begin religious observance again once they have children, and we were no different, although the ways in which we did this were considerably different from the ways in which we ourselves had been raised. Our sons were baptized in our living room by the priest who married us, with a blessing at the end sung by a female rabbi for whom I had been a dorm counselor in college. (Immediately after the Hebrew words died down, my father launched into a full-throated rendition of "When Irish Eyes Are Smiling," which he has always contended was in no way a protest against the rabbi.) We were so appalled by the limited theological knowledge of the parishioner who tutored us before our daughter's more traditional church christening that my husband, a former altar boy, provided the classes that led to Communion for each child: the prospective communicant would share the two-hour car ride from country to city on Sunday evenings, there on Route 80 to learn the seven sacraments, the names of the evangelists, and other factoids that would have enabled any of our three to score in the high 700s on a Catholicism SAT. We left it up to them whether to continue on to Confirmation, a consecration to the Church that we both felt was too important to be decided by us alone. None of the three has been confirmed.

"I told them I was a self-educated Catholic," Quin told us after an admissions interview at a Catholic boys' school, and the two of us, whipped into shape, and doctrine, by a procession of women in wimples and men in Roman collars, looked at each other sidelong: bet that went over like Bermuda shorts at Sunday Mass.

Today, of course, we see Bermuda shorts at Sunday Mass all the time. Which is an outrage, although not a religious one. It's hard to believe God has any interest in how we dress, and the only religious outrages are those of bigotry and hatred, like the right-wing evangelicals who protest military funerals with signs that say GOD HATES FAGS or the Muslim extremists who took down the World Trade Center and a corner of the Pentagon. Bermuda shorts in church are merely a sartorial sin.

Church garb was a major part of childhood observance for me, the modest dress, the hat, eventually the mantilla of Kennedy's Camelot and Vatican II. And perhaps, in retrospect, that signaled one of the inherent problems with the Catholic Church in which I grew to maturity. There was so much emphasis on form over faith, so much about head coverings and fish on Fridays and rote memorization. The lips moved but the mind was not engaged. Occasionally someone would make the argument that this was the foundation that would enable us to learn more, to think harder, to begin to appreciate the spiritual sense that was the point of the exercise. And yet, as far as I can see, that rarely happened. A small cadre of intellectual Catholics delved into the nature of God, of Christ, of the Gospels, of the soul and life after death. Sadly, many of those found themselves in trouble. Delving leads to questioning, and questioning leads to dissent, and dissent leads to disenfranchisement. "Every day a little closer to excommunication," my husband once said of my columns about the Church.

This is not just the lot of Catholics. Few religions foster a searching approach to spirituality. Piety has always found its most comfortable home in America amid newer immigrants, who welcome the shape devotion gives to an uncertain existence and the solace the spiritual provides in times of dislocation and want. But the more people are educated, the more they are skeptical; the more they are prosperous, the less likely they are to slavishly adhere to the faith of their fathers. In this way our family is a reflection of many others. Our grandparents were devout, our parents observant. And we are haphazard.

It's not that I've renounced the Church, although during the course of my lifetime it has provided so many reasons to do so. As other faiths have concluded that the Christ of the New Testament was a friend to women despite the strictures of his time and would have wanted them to lead and serve, the Catholic Church has been determined to marginalize its female members by denying them, with the flimsiest of arguments, the right to serve as priests. It has persisted in practicing a kind of theological gynecology by obsessing about contraception and abortion during a time of worldwide poverty and growing women's rights. It has cast in shadow the enormous contributions of righteous religious workers throughout the world by minimizing the scandal of pedophilia and other sexual predation that turns out to have been widespread in the Church.

That last was why I finally stopped putting on a skirt and heels each Sunday and going with my husband to Mass. I felt that my very presence in the pew suggested that I was willing to overlook the priests who had been shuffled from parish to parish, fondling children and teenagers as they went. But I'm not sure that was the only reason I stopped attending church. It's simply that, as I've grown older, I've had more time to think about the layers and layers of truth and understanding that make up the strata of our own personal earth. When they say there are no atheists in foxholes, the presumption is that the closer we come to mortality, the closer we will be to God. For me it has been the opposite. I was raised on stories and traditions. I know the lives of many saints, not just Thérèse and Bernadette, and the Sign of the Cross is so deeply ingrained in me that I have found it difficult not to use it in synagogues. Perhaps because of this, stories and symbols have become the basis of my professional life and the traditions of my family life. All five of us have assigned seats at the dinner table; woe betide the visitor who plops down in Chris's chair.

Our Christmases are vast inviolate repositories of custom: the Santa dolls on the mantel, the evergreen garland around the stair rail, the areas of the living room designated for the presents of each child although the children are now adults. Every year we go to the circus together, have done for decades. Each year we take up our bowls and spatulas and bake: oatmeal cookies for Quin, Toll House cookies for Maria, fudge for Chris, sugar cookies that the three of them will decorate with royal icing. The year that I believed Quin would be spending Christmas at his apartment in China almost did me in. He was a vegetarian at the time, and I wept in front of the veggie burger display at the supermarket as Muzak carols played on the PA system. When a group of Maria's friends showed up one evening on the sidewalk to sing carols and the Santa at the back took off his white beard to reveal himself as our eldest child, it was the clos-est I've ever come to fainting. My husband still considers flying Quin home from Beijing for Christmas among his cleverest pieces of subterfuge, and I consider it the nicest.

Every year, as a family, we read aloud Charles Dickens's *A Christmas Carol*. Neither my husband nor I can recall precisely how the tradition began, although we know we started it before we had children and then watched as, one by one, each learned to read well enough to manage an entire chapter, managed the pronunciation of words like "excrescence" and "apoplectic opu-lence." Learning to walk, learning to read, going to school, graduating from college—one of the notable markers of matu-rity in our family is having your own stave, or chapter, to read in the book. And because sometimes heaven is merciful, there are five staves, and five of us.

This should not be the centerpiece of the holiday. The birth of Christ should be the centerpiece. Actually, any good Catholic of a certain age can tell you that Easter ought to be so rather than Christmas, because this is when the promise of the Resurrection was fulfilled with a rolled-back stone and an empty tomb and the guarantee of life everlasting. But over the years Christmas has assumed a position of primal importance in our household, and the words of Charles Dickens in his slender novella have taken on the force of doctrine. I have quoted from that book in my own work more often than any other. "Are there no prisons?" Scrooge asks disdainfully of provisions for the poor. "Are there no workhouses?" And when the scales are lifted from his eyes by ghostly apparitions of the past, present, and future, those words are thrown back at him, and he, too, is made to understand that if you have two cloaks, you should give one to he who is shivering and in need. Dickens's tale makes me understand what it means to be a good person, just as the New Testament has.

I've thought of my faith so often as I've grown older, and I admit that I'm not certain what I really believe about any of it anymore. And, frankly, I'm not sure it matters. If the message of Christ led me to try to be a more generous human being, does it matter whether he was the Messiah or a prophet? If people are empathetic and charitable, does it matter whether they believe in a God who somehow began, or engineered, or oversees us all? If we have traded the evangelists for Dickens, is that a tragedy or a draw? Those questions take me far, far away from the positions of the Church in which I was baptized and the beliefs I had many years ago, and into the realm of humanism, secularism, even heresy.

I don't say that with the gleeful "gotcha" of the dedicated atheist or the cynical dismissal of the enthusiastically lapsed Catholic—recovering Catholics, some of them call themselves. Atheism is a game for younger people, who are so sure of what they're sure of. Contempt for religion and for Catholicism (as opposed to contempt for the men who poorly lead the Church) makes me breathless and ill at ease; a smug certitude about the foolishness of a point of view that has been held for millennia by such bright lights as Saint Augustine, Thomas More, C. S. Lewis, and Graham Greene just seems silly. But the writings and beliefs of those great men intrigue yet do not entirely persuade. I am less sure of what I know than of those things of which I'm doubtful.

When I coach students through essay writing, I invariably give the most able the same direction: go deeper, go deeper. In each iteration, reveal more, of who you truly are, of what you really think. That's the hallmark of aging, too, that we learn to go deeper, in our friendships, in our family life, in our reflections on how we live and how we face the future. The reason we develop an equanimity about our lives and ourselves is that we have gone deep into what has real meaning.

And the mark, I suppose, of an indelible connection to religious faith is that ability to go deeper, to burrow into the self, to expand spiritual connections and limitations. I'm stuck too close to the surface. Perhaps that is because of my own shortcomings. Perhaps it has something to do with the fact that I was raised in a Church that does not invite its people to go deeper, or to move very far beyond its outward forms. Catholicism is an autocracy. It not only dismisses questioning, it demonizes it. The tiny subclass of Catholics who bring deep intellectual rigor to issues of tradition, doctrine, infallibility, identity, and sanctity are almost always honored in the breach if they are honored at all. The price for that is that many of the faithful, especially highly educated ones, either skate on the surface or fall away.

At some level I may have lost my religion, despite the deep talons of its traditions and forms within me. But I've never lost, and will never lose, my faith. "Faith is the substance of things hoped for, the evidence of things not seen," it says in the book of Hebrews. I believe in hope and mystery. That belief is just different than it once was. I remember being mesmerized as a child by the fact that one indication that Bernadette was truly blessed by God was that her body had not decomposed, that you could travel to Lourdes and see her, in her nun's habit, a rosary entwined in her waxy hands, lying in an elaborate glass coffin. Having now seen Mao Tse-tung and Lenin in a similar state, that seems like a cheap parlor trick to me, beneath the dignity of an uneducated woman who either saw visions or was brave enough to insist she had. I look at the list of miracles that earned Thérèse a place at the table of sainthood, and they're poor narrow things, all about illness and ailments, tuberculosis and arthritis and cancer allegedly cured.

By those standards radiation is miraculous, and antibiotics. Actually, by any standards those are miracles. And there are all those little everyday miracles, too, the fact that a daffodil bulb sprouts a flower year after year, that kittens know to use a litter box without being taught, that the music of Samuel Barber and Stephen Sondheim and the last sentences of *A Christmas Carol* make your soul rise and shine. "God bless us, every one," the book ends. I trust He does.

Step Aside

When I was a young reporter I went to Key West one
Easter weekend to interview Tennessee Williams,
who was chipper, voluble, and fascinating in the
mornings and then became progressively less so as the day
waned and he had more and more to drink. There was no mystery about the source of the profound sadness that came over
him as night fell. It was the genius version of sundown syndrome; he suspected, feared, in fact knew that he would never
again write anything like *The Glass Menagerie* or *A Streetcar
Named Desire,* both produced when he was in his thirties. It was
a kind of journalistic malpractice to expect a twenty-five-year-
old reporter to understand this; there surely must have been
something in this courtly man that recoiled from my youthful
get-up-and-go. I cringe now at the memory of the great men
who opened their doors to what they can only have concluded
was the most callow and clueless of interviewers: John Ashbery
explaining his epic poem *Self-Portrait in a Convex Mirror,* Rich-
ard Yates talking about his great novel *Revolutionary Road.* But

they were all so lovely to me, Williams especially; he let me wear a sun hat he said had belonged to his beloved sister, Rose, the model for Laura in *Menagerie*.

I've thought of that weekend often as I've watched some of my colleagues become accomplished, well known, even famous, as they became people with power and influence. It's interesting to see what happens as those you've known as ambitious kids age and prosper. The best are the ones who don't forget the rungs on the ladder, who remember what it was like to climb, the ones who believe it is almost a moral requirement to be generous to the young, as Williams was to me. Sure, it can feel like being replaced, or embalmed, when the new generation of strivers shows up. But one of the best and most dignified opportunities to stay engaged in the world as you grow older is to give a hand to those who come after. Rise up, reach down. Of course, what that means is that at a certain point you have to step aside. Jump, or be pushed; it's as simple as that.

I remember judging an award for reporters under the age of thirty-five some years ago, when I was a columnist at *Newsweek* and trying to decide how much longer to stay in the job. As I paged through the contest entries I couldn't help noticing the dates. One talented reporter was born the year I graduated from college, another just about the time I arrived at *The New York Times,* one when I was covering City Hall, another when I was writing my first column.

Needless to say, this made me feel really old. But it also made me think about the conundrum the baby boom has created for our kids, and our country. Born between 1946 and 1964, boomers take up more room than any other generation in American history. And so, inevitably, we have created a kind of bottleneck, in the professions, in politics, in power. The frustration this poses for the young and talented should be obvious. In my personal life it was reflected indelibly on the day when, talking of the unwillingness of many of my friends to retire, my eldest child noted, "You guys just won't go."

When my parents were my son's age, there was an orderliness to how one generation moved aside and another stepped up to primacy and prosperity. It was reflected in life expectancy, in the fact that most American males, those who comprised most of the workforce, lived only a few years past the statutory retirement age of sixty-five.

Even when I was the same age as my children are now, there was a natural transition from one generation to another. Every year a small group of reporters would retire and leave the newsroom, to be replaced by younger ones. (With the harsh insensitivity of youth I thought this was perfectly fine.) In many businesses this rite of passage is disappearing, and the number of people who work into their seventies and eighties has climbed steadily over the last two decades. There are some professions that still have mandatory retirement, but the number has dwindled. Forcing someone to retire at sixty-five simply feels different when life expectancy is eighty. How many stories have you heard about the guy who died of a heart attack three months after someone gave him an engraved watch and a handshake? What was with the watch, anyhow? *Tick tick tick,* nowhere to go, no place to be. One study showed that more than one out of every ten members of the federal bench is over age eighty. Another study may show why: more than nine out of ten district court judges die within a year of retiring fully. As Susan B. Anthony once said, "I don't want to die as long as I can work; the minute I cannot, I want to go."

The retirement parties I've attended always had an underlying pathos, the feeling that groomsmen seem to have at a wedding: thank God it's not me up there. Dan Gilbert, a psychology professor at Harvard who studies happiness, has said that one of the most traumatic experiences in the human span of life is unemployment. And retirement the way we once defined retirement is pretty much unemployment with a party beforehand. Everyone talks about it as though it's this great luxury, this incredible gift, to do nothing all day, to throw away the alarm clock and the calendar, to make it up as it comes. They say that it's such a shame that people can't afford to retire these days, or not until they're too old to enjoy it. But I'm not convinced. I remember the old guys who manned the chairs at the barbershop my father used to visit, and the stooped and ashen bartender at a place he took me for pizza when I'd been a particularly good girl. The older man who still worked behind the counter with his sons at the butcher shop where I bought meat when my kids were young wasn't there because he liked getting the veal thinner than a sheet of shirt cardboard but because the customers, the banter, the outslicing the sons—that was his life.

For women today, retirement sometimes means being downsized from two jobs simultaneously. For years I was doing two full-time jobs during one full-time life. I took three kids in the car or on the train to school, ran back to the house, grabbed coffee and dropped into a desk chair, wrote until mid-afternoon, and went back to pick the kids up again. I basically worked as a mother between three P.M. and nine A.M., and as a writer between nine and three. Today I still write between nine and three, even though I am the parent of three college graduates who all have driver's licenses and MetroCards and can get themselves wherever they need to go. At the same time that I am doing somewhat less in my work life, I am doing much less in my mom life as well.

But that doesn't really have to mean less, just different. I had breakfast with an old friend, Michele Tolela Myers, who has been an academic, an administrator, and finally the president of two liberal arts colleges, Denison and Sarah Lawrence. If she wanted to write "The End" at the bottom of her résumé right now, it would still be very impressive. But when she was a young woman, balancing real life and big dreams, the dream she'd left behind was to be a novelist. And she's writing novels now. Perhaps one of the most significant aspects of our longer life expectancy is that we have time for a half-life, a quarter-life, in which, if we're courageous and strategic, we can make that sort of unrealized dream come true.

Now, there's no point in idealizing this. For every dream deferred and then pursued, there's someone whose dream was to work in perpetuity at a job as out of reach as youth. For every person who gladly continues to work, there is another forced back into a workplace he thought he'd earned the right to leave, dragged out of bed and into the car by a sharp drop in savings or pension. For every person who believes she's gotten a chance at a third act, there is one who feels cast aside.

As a fiction writer, I know that one of the key questions of the form is "What happens next?" When Charles Dickens's novel *The Old Curiosity Shop* was being released, chapter by chapter, in serial form, crowds famously lined the waterfront in New York to shout at a ship arriving from London, "Is Little Nell dead?" But it's not only in fictional plot that the question is central but also in our own lives. What happens next? Over the years academics have measured the transition from child to adult by five markers: finishing school, moving out of your parents' home, becoming financially independent of them, getting married, and having kids. One of the biggest differences between my father's generation and that of my children is that fifty years ago the majority of men and women had checked off all those milestones by age thirty, while today the number who have done so by that same age has dwindled significantly, in young men to below a third. My parents at twenty-five were married, had two children, and owned their first home courtesy of the low-interest mortgage my father earned through his stint in the military. At twenty-five my husband and I were newly married; we bought our first home a year later but wouldn't have our first child until we were thirty-one. At twenty-five my children envision both marriage and home ownership in the future, perhaps a somewhat distant one. Many of the big things haven't happened for them yet.

For those who punched all those tickets early, a different problem arises, not of maturity postponed but of maturity unvarying. One problem with aging is that we fear nothing much will happen next, that the plot points have passed. At a certain juncture, the hand you've been dealt is the entire deck. Some of us will marry again, even have second families. But while the early decades were punctuated with graduations, weddings, promotions, relocations, there comes that moment when all we can do is redecorate. If nothing happens in the story of our lives, is it even a story at all? Or what if the only things that happen are bad things, one loss after another?

Take away work, and for many the vista can be grim. That may be why the old retirement model of the lounge chair and the golf cart could be gone for good. Women may provide an alternate model of a more active and involved retirement that is more consonant with the way we live now. Those women trying to balance work and family have been agitating for years for part-time and flex-time work hours; what better arrangement for older workers who carry institutional memory but want less of the load? Those women who decided not to work for a time after their children were born often used their skills for volunteer projects; what better use for the talents of those of us who want to be busy but don't necessarily need a salary?

During our lifetime, women's lives have been about redefinition, over and over and over again, while men's lives are still often about maintaining the status quo. But aging is not a status quo situation. It seems that men may have to learn to live more like us, particularly in their later years. No doubt some will have to be dragged kicking and screaming into our newly configured world and out of their linear thinking in which a person climbs the career ladder until he dies, will have to be persuaded that a lateral move may be satisfying as well as necessary.

We all need a Plan B. I know this very well. I'm a person who is never going to be playing golf. My prejudice against golf is one of those silly unreasonable prejudices that all of us acquire from time to time, that are really an attempt at self-important self-definition. Sometimes these prejudices are destructive, like unreasonable dislikes of ethnic or racial groups. Sometimes they're pretty benign, like saying you aren't willing to taste raw fish even if it's billed as sushi. Bait, my father calls it, but he's a pretty unadventurous eater: steak, spaghetti, grilled cheese sandwiches, Tastykake cupcakes. The only weird food he eats is something called scrapple that you fry up for breakfast.

My father doesn't play golf, either. He mainly reads now, although he used to fish. I used to fish, too. But even though I like to fish, I couldn't fish full time, couldn't pack it in and go down to the beach and surf cast in the mornings and then while away the rest of the day at tackle shops and marinas. I'm happy to settle for less, but not for nothing at all.

About a decade ago a financial guy had my husband and me lined up on the other side of his desk, and he asked what our plans for retirement might be. I imagine Gerry had the same look on his face that I had, the look usually described colloquially as "being hit over the head with a board," because the financial guy said quickly, "Oh, you're those people." Yep, we are. You know those mellow young people who spend months taking trains across Europe, knock around wondering what they're going to do next, hopscotch from one thing to another, unapologetically seeking passion, direction, vocation? We were never those people. In my case, I suspect it's part of my essential metabolism. One of my favorite photographs was taken when I was about two years old. There's a lot to love: my mother's old-fashioned swing jacket, disguising what from personal experience I suspect is a baby belly; my father's sharp young fifties'-dad look, complete with professorial glasses; the fact that I'm wearing those matching wool leggings with my dress coat that were de rigueur and uncomfortably itchy. Daddy is holding my brother Bob, a sack of flour in a blanket, while my mother is bent slightly with her arm outstretched to pull Anna back into the Happy Family formation. That little girl is taking off. It's a still photograph, of course, but you can almost feel it—places to go, people to see, legs to pump, legs probably less than a foot long.

There are two ways that kind of hyperdrive kid can go in later life: either her push-push finds no place to put itself and drives her wild, or it finds an object and the object finds her back. I was lucky to go the second way, hectoring an editor into giving me a copy girl's job, making a world out of words.

I had lunch with a young reporter one day, and her description of her week was like Proust's madeleine, or a whiff of the cigars my father once smoked. In an instant in my mind there was a world complete: the editor, the assignment, the subway ride, the street full of strangers telling the story or turning their backs at the sight of the notebook and the pen, the subway ride, the phone calls, the story, the editors, the truncated version on an inside page. Lather, rinse, repeat the next day, and the next, until the bottom drawer of my desk was lousy with notebooks with random scribbles in different colors of pen. The very notion gives me a shot of adrenaline. And then I feel exhausted. There has to be a middle ground between bouncing around Brooklyn looking for old Dodgers fans for a feature story and tormenting my children with text messages because I'm unemployed. Maybe the new model for retirement is some middle ground.

Certainly for many of us the old model just won't suit. Until recently, given the male monolith in the work world, retirement was a guy's business, and no matter how people pretend otherwise, it was grim. My experience is that guys like routine, and most of them had it: shower, shave, dress or uniform shirt, brief-case or tools, car, office, work work work, home for dinner. To suddenly expect such a man, after forty years, to putter around the house and flip the channels from his comfy chair borders on sadism. It's also no fun for his stay-at-home wife, who had her own routine: dishes, vacuum, coffee, sandwich, telephone, Oprah, cooking. A big bestseller at flea markets is a plaque that shows what that kind of woman thinks of her husband's retire-ment: I TOOK HIM FOR BETTER OR FOR WORSE, BUT NOT FOR LUNCH.

In the face of this, many of my fellow boomers have vowed to fight aging, and downsizing, to the death. I take their point about experience and wisdom in the workplace. I joined the en-tire nation, the day that Chesley Sullenberger landed a passen-ger jet safely on the Hudson River, in thanking God that a man who had been flying for a lifetime and a crew of veteran flight attendants had been working that afternoon.

But there's another side to that equation as well, and younger workers see it, and resent it, and for good reason. If no one steps aside, there is no room for advancement. The pipeline is clogged and sluggish without the vitality that new blood brings. It's par-ticularly glaring when this generational stall happens in the news business, which constantly remakes itself in the image and likeness of the world. What an incredible time it was to grow up in that business! My first stories were written on typewriters, with carbon paper, my last with a computer that emailed my copy to the desk. I called in breaking news from phone booths; one of my young colleagues just showed me a story she'd writ-ten with her thumbs on her BlackBerry. It was a good story, too.

I was bereft when Brenda Starr, the flame-haired comic-strip character with the starry eyes who convinced me (incor-rectly) as a child that newspaper work was glamorous, handed in her notebook and passed out of existence just as she turned seventy. But I accept that journalism will have to keep changing as the world changes. It's not like the old ways were so wonderful: read the *Times,* or any local daily, on microfilm from the fifties or sixties, and you will immediately see how narrow daily journalism was, how boring the writing, how in the tank for business interests and political authority it could be. There is nothing quite as tedious, or as useless, as ritual recitations of the good old days, which in many ways weren't.

Our lifetime has been such a time of change, in the economy, in education, in politics, in the work world. But no one seems eager to change on an individual level, to make way for fresh perspectives and new ideas. That linear path, the ladder, emphasizes stability, but too often at the expense of innovation and mobility. Since the day the youthful John F. Kennedy delivered his inaugural address, when I was eight years old, people have been quoting his saying that the torch had been passed to a new generation. But torches don't really get passed very much; people love to hold on to them.

We give way to the young not simply because it is right but because it is both inevitable and desirable: Dickens to George Eliot, Faulkner to Philip Roth. Something in the human heart, something we try to quell when it interferes with our own comfort, nevertheless calls out: Next! That's what I heard when I was judging that contest, when I read those young reporters' stories. It was a message delivered without rancor or contempt, the same one I'd heard from my own son: It's our turn. Step aside.

Mortality

At first it was just a dress. I bought it one day in late August at the little dress shop I like near our house in the country, the one where they know I'll never wear cargo pants or anything with sequins. It was black, and well cut without being chic, made from one of those new miracle fabrics that never wrinkle even after three hours of riding with your torso in the half nelson of a seat belt. There's a certain sort of dress you find in fashion magazines that's kind of nothing, really; the editors get two pages out of showing you how to dress it up with a belt and a brooch or dress it down with boots and a cardigan. This is that kind of dress. It took me a couple of days to realize it was something else as well. It was the perfect funeral dress.

We all wind up there eventually, first in fits and starts, then precipitously, so that the memorial services and shiva calls and sympathy notes begin to blur, to seem like some continuous loop of murmured condolences and black clothes. LIFE'S A BITCH, says the T-shirt, AND THEN YOU DIE. So glib, because that's not the problem at all. Life's great, and then you die. And, perhaps as important, the others do first.

The world shrinks. Someone once told me the answer is to make young friends, but that's not the answer. The thing about old friends is not that they love you but that they know you. They remember that disastrous New Year's Eve when you mixed White Russians and champagne, and how you wore that red maternity dress until everyone was sick of seeing the blaze of it in the office, and the uncomfortable couch in your first apartment, and the smoky stove in your beach rental. They look at you and don't really think you look older, because they've grown old along with you, and, like the faded paint in a beloved room, they're used to the look. And then one of them is gone, and you've lost a chunk of yourself. The stories of the terrorist attacks of 2001, the tsunami, the Japanese earthquake, always used numbers, the deaths of thousands a measure of how great the disaster. Catastrophe is numerical. Loss is singular, one beloved at a time.

Everyone knows this is coming, especially someone with a history like mine. I was old enough neither to rent a car nor to score a college diploma when I was made to understand, indelibly and unequivocally, as my mother dwindled away and then went out like a pale candle, that without much warning, good people die, losing what was left of their span, leaving those who love them to soldier on with unending pain and loss.

That is ultimately the point of all this, isn't it? When we talk about aging, we talk about flagging libido, increasing infirmities, being passed over at work, being bored at home. But the elephant in the room is mortality. It's death, but no one likes to speak his name, as though to acknowledge is to conjure, and to conjure is to invite him into the house. We speak of mammograms and cholesterol and calorie counts and we pretend what we are discussing is health, diet, appearance, vigor. But under it all is the shadow that never goes away.

I met mortality up close and personal on January 18, 1972, when I was nineteen years old and my mother, whose birth name was Prudence Marguerite Pantano, had barely entered her forties. Although she had done everything possible to avoid the hospital, she died there. For the wake they had to fill in with tissue paper the bodice of the black-and-white print dress that she liked so much because it had belonged to her when she was a more robust woman, plumper, more zaftig. In one of the cruel ironies of these episodes, she had dwindled to a narrow reed of a person with a round, hard, protuberant belly. It was her belief that she was pregnant that took her to the doctor in the first place, and during the last months of her illness that was exactly how she appeared. A woman who had spent the best years of her life in maternity clothes, she sickened and died in them as well. I made her dresses on the Singer sewing machine I had been given as a gift for my sixteenth birthday. The one made of navy dotted swiss was the one she liked best. It was cheery.

In the same fashion that she asked for wall-to-wall carpeting for Christmas while my father preferred to buy her jewelry or cashmere, her wishes for those final months were humdrum and domestic. She liked the two of us to go to lunch at some small restaurant where they served salads and soups. She wanted to stay up and watch movies on the *Late Late Show: Wuthering Heights, Waterloo Bridge, All About Eve, A Place in the Sun.* (For years I was the only person I knew who was conversant with Carole Lombard's plane crash while she was on a war-bonds tour and the long friendship between Elizabeth Taylor and Montgomery Clift.) She sat in the kitchen in her wheelchair and taught me to cook, mostly things I still make for my family today, tomato sauce and meatballs, meatloaf with a latticework of bacon on top, chicken Parmigiano.

I would like to portray myself as the little heroine of this story, but it would be a lie so terrible that, even no longer believing in heaven or hell—though I wish I did, at least the former—

I feel as though I would be struck down for it. I did not want to be there. I felt powerless, trapped, enfeebled. This had less to do with my mother, whom I loved, than with the life she and her cohort had lived, which terrified me. I was afraid of the briars of housewifery turning me into a Sleeping Beauty, taking away Doris Lessing and Simone de Beauvoir and leaving me with *Joy of Cooking,* Jacqueline Susann, and slipcovers.

When my daughter was nineteen she wrote to me that she could scarcely believe she was the age at which I had taken over the house and the children, the pain management and the hospital visits. But I didn't take them over so much as live through them. And above all I didn't open the door into the dark spiritual tunnel in which my mother must have been living much of the time. Perhaps if I had she would have politely shut it in my face. We do what we can to protect our children from pain, even if it means we shoulder it ourselves. "If you want help, you shouldn't act like a person who never needs any," my daughter muttered to me one night when I was angry, and for once I was at a loss for words because she had so completely nailed my modus operandi.

My mother was a variation on this theme of the sacrificial mother. She always took the smallest and most sinewy piece of chicken, the burnt edge of the baked ziti. My husband's family had a dinner table code I'd never heard before: FHB, or Family Hold Back. My mother always made so much food that the issue didn't arise among us, but if it had, the code would have been MHB, and she would have. There's a line in the classic Jean Shepherd movie *A Christmas Story* in which the narrator says of his own family, "My mother had not had a hot meal for herself in fifteen years." I never found it funny, simply true. The habit of self-sacrifice was so deeply ingrained in my mother's character that she even protected strangers from discomfort. Once, waiting for chemo, she told another woman that she was at the hospital because she'd broken her arm.

"Now you'll have something to write about," she said one afternoon in the kitchen, apropos of nothing, talking without talking at all about the terrible thing that was happening to her as, instead, a terrible thing that was happening to me. I knew her, although not as well as I wish I had, or as I've known her in retrospect, as the freelance archaeologist of her past, and I can tell you that there was nothing malicious in that comment, that all she wanted to say was that something good could come out of bad. But in the years afterward it echoed within me because of the appalling suggestion that I could only be generous if there was something in it for me, if I came out of the experience with some material, something I could use.

She left me her engagement ring. When I was twenty-three someone broke into my apartment and stole it along with all my other jewelry. "Do you know how big it was?" the police officer said. "Not big," I said.

She wanted to live. That was the lesson I learned from her. She wanted to live until she decided she didn't. It's true of us all. We put fences around that property: I wouldn't want to live if I were in pain. I wouldn't want to live if I had that disease, this cancer. And then, miraculously, we're in pain, with that disease, this cancer, and we want to live still. There's always another threshold.

I don't know how we're expected to think of this. Sometimes I power walk along the Hudson, the park to my left, the river to my right, the smoggy absence in the skyline where the World Trade Center towers once stood, then smoked, burned, fell, and I think that someday the river will run, the trees leaf out, the blue sky vibrate overhead, the runners pound out the miles on the path, the dog walkers throw their balls, the nannies push the strollers, but I will not be there. I will be gone. It reminds me of the truculent way in which, when small, my daughter used to look at photographs of her two brothers at the beach or at their birthday parties before her arrival. The idea of a time before she was born, before she existed, before we knew her and were required to have her in our daily lives for our happiness and sense of completion, a time when Quin and Chris were alive without her—it did not strike her as strange or even unimaginable but as an outrage, an insult. She couldn't wrap her mind around it. Why should she?

Once my mother was gone, I was left trying to wrap my mind around the fact that death was always lurking. It was difficult, returning to college, going about the ordinary life of a twenty-year-old, which is as removed from mortality as it is from the kind of domestic responsibility that had become second nature to me. There was suddenly an unseen barrier between me and nearly everyone else. I knew the secret that was not a secret, that the molecules of the living world are always rearranging themselves so that something is lost, something is lost every day.

My friends discovered it little by little, over the years. The conversations over the phone in a low register began, one by one: Oh, did you hear about so-and-so? So tragic, so unexpected, so young. But I never felt that it was unexpected, or that anyone was young. I felt the weight of knowledge. For years I felt that my mother had lived to a fairly substantial age, until the passage of time and my own maturity taught me first that she had died very young indeed and then that she had been robbed of fully half her existence.

There was a period when I became less alone in this knowledge of mortality, the sad period during the 1980s when many of us began to watch our gay friends waste away, when we first learned about AIDS and its fine points, T cell counts, antivirals. Every few months there was a name to add to the list, and then medical advances and the activism of the gay community beat back death. Safe sex became commonplace and AIDS became a chronic condition instead of a black flag, and the deaths of young men began to slow. And then the breast cancer began, and the early heart attacks. Yet for many the denial continued. How often have I attended memorial services for men about whom their friends said that they really began to understand what mattered when they got the diagnosis? There's simply no excuse for that, no matter what the average life expectancy, no matter how good modern medicine. The simple exigencies and experiences of life should teach us what life is all about. To not get the message without a cancer diagnosis, a hand tremor, a pain in the left side of the chest, is just foolishness.

Generations before us were not taken aback by death, early or otherwise. Epidemics, infant mortality, incurable illnesses, wars, disasters: survival was a gift. The heart stopped. The breathing ceased. And it did so often. Flu and smallpox and measles, illnesses we scarcely register, sent millions to early graves. And the wars started, and the soldiers left and never came back. Existence was often short and brutish. Without antibiotics or reliable surgery, prayer was their only solace.

But with the development of the respirator, the feeding tube, in vitro fertilization, frozen embryos, the question of what actually constitutes life became not only germane but infinitely complex. Because of all that we've learned and all that we can do, we may be the first generation of human beings who try to deny our own mortality. The great Catholic writer Thomas Merton wrote in his journal, "Never has man's helplessness in the face of death been more pitiable than in this age when he can do everything except escape death." There is a story about Jacqueline Kennedy Onassis, maybe apocryphal, although I hope not. It is said that when she was diagnosed, in her early sixties, with lymphoma, she responded, "If I had known this was going to happen, I wouldn't have done all those sit-ups."

It is going to happen. The light at the end of the tunnel, as the poet Robert Lowell once wrote, is the light of an oncoming train. We know this and yet, like the little girl who refuses to acknowledge the possibility of a world without her skipping through it, our minds cannot accept it fully. But the gift that some of us have been given, in exchange for terrible loss, is the gift of that knowledge. My mother thought her death would enrich my writing, and I'm ashamed to say that she was correct in that.

One day my son and I were talking about an interview with his college writing professor in which she had said that she believed most writers had only one subject. "Well, Mom, if you only have one subject, yours is motherhood," he said offhandedly. I found his insight reassuring, and cheering, yet I couldn't help editing it mentally: motherhood, and loss. That's what I write about most often.

But it actually was on my character that my mother's death made the most indelible mark. It made me certain that life was short, and therefore it made me both driven and joyful. I couldn't waste time and I couldn't take anything for granted, couldn't be jaded or bored. Call it a cliché, but one of my favorite moments in theater is Emily Webb's monologue from beyond the grave in *Our Town*. She looks around at the living and cries, "Oh, earth, you're too wonderful for anybody to realize you. Do any human beings ever realize life while they live it?— every, every minute?"

Those of us who have lost a parent young are a particular breed. My friend David was one, too, his doctor father dead at fifty-three of a heart attack, which is why he took such good care of himself, exercising, eating well. The morning he was walking his dog toward Central Park and felt a weight in his chest, he took a cab to the hospital and was in surgery within hours. With me it was the annual pelvic sonograms and, finally, the ovariectomy. We knew exactly where to look for bad news. But of course while you're looking to the right, something can sneak up on your left, which is what happened when David died in a car accident.

Once we were talking, I remember, about what we called the magic number. It is the age to which your parent lived. When I had outlived my mother I looked at every year, every passage, every event, the way the early explorers must have looked at the islands of the new world. "I felt like every year was a gift," David said, and we both nodded. And for all of those years his refrain was this: "Aren't we lucky?"

It is inevitable that watching your mother die at a young age will make you feel like the last of your line. Your mother is, quite literally, where you come from. It never escaped even my dim-witted nineteen-year-old notice that the place in her pelvis that killed Prudence Quindlen was the place where I'd lived for nine months before I arrived, large and covered with lanugo hair, so that the poor woman cried at how strange I looked. I wonder who thought to tell me about those tears? It wasn't her. She hated when I mentioned it. She was afraid it would reinforce the faint unspoken schism between us, the quiet and gentle mother, the extroverted and ebullient daughter.

But I'm not the last of the line. I am the mother of my mother's grandchildren. That made the hard lesson I'd learned early on easier, and more distressing, too. It meant that she lived on in those three children, with their dark dark eyes, brown-black like hers, not green like my own. But it meant, too, that I knew I might not live on with them. My sister was nine years old when our mother died, and she remembers nothing. Nothing. Sometimes I mention something, about a dress our mother wore, about a dish she made, about how she brushed and braided our thick brown hair. And Theresa says, "Really?" and it breaks my heart.

Sometimes when Quin was five and Chris was three, when Quin was eight and Chris six and Maria three, when they were all the world to me, I would look at them and think of my sister, of how she couldn't remember how our mother sounded or looked, and say to myself, I don't even really count for these children yet. If I die tomorrow they will have nothing but other people's stories where a mother ought to be.

This is why I sometimes haven't felt about aging the way my friends have, why I was thrilled to be forty, happy at fifty, why I don't dread sixty or even seventy. I'm elated to have what the actress Laura Linney called "the privilege of aging." I'm living for two, for all the years, the decades, my mother never got. I'm storing up memories, not for me but for my kids, so that they will have a cache greater than my own.

Not long ago I trawled the basement and the bookshelves and pulled together for each of them a complete set of my books. When they asked, I said I just wanted to be certain that there was a copy of each book for each of them. Maybe they were fooled, but I wasn't fooling myself. Life everlasting, in hardcover.

It would be a great solace to believe in life after death, but I no longer do. Perhaps it is because of having seen a person die, that shocking moment when an individual becomes essentially an object. The bird has flown. Only the cage remains.

I once had a nun who posited that the afterlife might consist largely of electrical impulses, free-floating personalities, that since matter could neither be created nor destroyed, brain waves would endure. "What kind of nuns taught you?" my husband asked, incredulous, when I told him that. But it made more sense than the heaven we'd been raised on. When I was six I took my first airplane flight and I looked for any sign of something above the clouds. Even then it seemed like a chancy proposition: if we would all be reunited, would that mean the great-uncle who unrelentingly mocked my thumb-sucking would be there, too?

When life on earth was hell, in the time of plagues, of starvation and slavery, the idea of another life, a better life, must have seemed both irresistible and necessary. And for the bereaved it provided solace. "She's at peace now," someone told me at my mother's wake. It's one of the only things I remember, that and the black dress with white polka dots I wore. Years later I was always surprised when this friend or that would say they had been there that day. I was in a fugue state, insensible, poised between the girl I had been and the woman I would become.

"She's in a better place," that same person said. I remember the dress, and the rage. There is no better place. This is the best place, here, now, alive, a chipmunk scampering across the stones, a cloud scudding across the sky, the dogs barking at nothing on the road, the road running empty into an unseen distance and beyond, my husband busy at the office, my children busy in the world. The better place is along the Hudson River, where the loon bobs on the swell from the ferry and dives for unseen fish until it seems he must drown, then pops up glistening twenty feet from where he went down. The better place is that spot on the highway when you can suddenly see New York City strung like a necklace of jagged diamonds, and that corner of the porch where the house wrens build their nest and then disassemble it and build it again, and the table at Thanksgiving and the tree at Christmas. My father persuaded my mother that she had to stay alive through Christmas, and after it was over, he said, "Easter comes early this year." And she said, "To hell with Easter," and was dead by mid-January.

I hate January. At the beginning of every new year I get a sinking sensation. All these years later, sometimes I think it's the lack of sunlight, or the unwavering cold. And then I remember. There are some things that are deep inside me now, chemical, biological: The way my head swivels when a little voice cries, "Mommy!" in a crowded supermarket. The adrenaline rush late on an election night. The anvil weight of January.

In *Angels in America,* the brilliant play by Tony Kushner, a play about illness and love and loss and death, there is this valediction: "But still. Still bless me anyway. I want more life. I can't help myself. I do." I do.

To Be Continued

There's a pond to one side of our house in the country. It is full of fish, most of them bought and paid for: bass, sunnies, trout, and the fat old grass carp that are supposed to keep the bottom vegetation in check. My son and I found a turtle on the banks with a freshwater leech and its dozens of young attached to the shell, so the pond must have leeches, too. I put a hundred catfish in the pond and haven't seen one since the hatchery truck drove away, except the one the young dog managed to catch and then couldn't manage to eat because of that spiny dorsal fin.

The pond is man-made but you'd never know it. The previous owner, who was a successful businessman but had the soul and the inclination of an engineer, designed it perfectly. At times of flood it remains precisely within its banks, and at times of drought it does the same. It is fed by five springs and disgorges into a narrow spillway that leads to Cherry Creek. The trees bud, leaf, drop their leaves, shiver in the winter wind; the shrubs bloom, go to seed, hunch beneath the snow. But the pond never changes. Sometimes if it's extremely cold in winter it will get a sheet of ice over the section near the dock, but the ice is never thick enough to walk on.

When we first looked at the place, the man who'd long taken care of it told us there was a bit of a heron problem. We thought that was hilarious, and amazing. A heron problem! We would see heron! How could that be a problem? Now I swear softly at them as they rise from the banks of the pond just after dawn, silver ghosts on stilt legs, spearing my fish.

When I'm here I walk around the perimeter of the pond two, sometimes three times a day. Early in our tenancy I imagined for just a moment that I saw a woman sitting in one of the Adirondack chairs at the far end. She had silver hair and was wearing nothing-colored clothes, a loose shirt and pants. At first I couldn't tell who she was. The only other woman I'd ever encountered unexpectedly on the property was the previous owner's wife, who had long outlived him and died at age ninety-one. After we had taken title but before we'd moved in, I had spent three days there alone, putting sheets on the beds, hanging pictures, placing towels, making the house my own. But I was sleeping in her old bedroom and using her beautiful old cherry desk, and the first night as I fell asleep I felt as though someone incorporeal was standing next to the bed. So I said very loudly, "Bess, this is my house now." And that was that.

I am not in the least the kind of person who believes in ghosts or vibrations or hauntings or visions. I wish I were; there are all sorts of people I would love to see again even if I could see through them. And the woman in the Adirondack chair wasn't someone who, in the parlance of spiritualists, had passed over. When I squinted at her I realized that she looked familiar, and the reason she looked familiar was that she looked like me, only much older. Then she was gone, and there was just a rain jacket that had been left draped across the chair and a tree branch at an odd angle behind it. It was all my overactive imagination. But frankly, for just an instant I thought I looked pretty good.

It's hard to imagine yourself in the future. It's why people do so many dumb things, because they're mired in the moment. Smoking, drinking, making disastrous marriages, putting off medical tests. The reason we've made a mess of the planet is that being its stewards required us to imagine not our own futures but those four or five generations removed. It's a quantum leap, from unthinkingly letting the water run into the drain as you brush your teeth to global shortages of water when your great-grandchildren are old people themselves. It's probably unimaginable in any concrete way.

"The human being is the only animal that thinks about the future," Daniel Gilbert wrote in his book, *Stumbling on Happiness*. But thinking about it is different from inhabiting it, or imagining it, or believing in it truly. Thinking about the future is how people come up with a route to the top job. Inhabiting it is how they realize the top job is an invitation to a coronary and a life of misery. The second mostly happens in real time.

It's not surprising to me that I can't really imagine what I will be like at eighty. I can't imagine myself at twenty. I know the anecdotes, the life passages, the résumé. But to feel what that girl felt, to close my eyes and actually be her: it's beyond me. Like one of those paintings on which artists have put several strata of fully realized compositions, there's simply been too much layered upon the way she was for me to see it clearly. I'm always amazed by people who can tell you precisely how they felt in first grade, at their junior prom. Sometimes I can tell you who was there, what I wore, the address of the house. The reporter remembers the facts: I grew up in a center-hall colonial at 511 Kenwood Road. When you walk in the front door, the living room is to the left, the dining room to the right. But the novelist cannot truly evoke the emotions, conjure the scene. Or she can, but has no idea whether it is accurate or merely imagined. Only ephemera makes the past seem somewhat real, poems written in my more rounded youthful script, photographs found in a drawer, a forgotten earring at the bottom of the jewelry box. So much of the rest is like a movie whose plot outline I recall but whose scenes I've mostly forgotten.

Sometimes I think we can't imagine our future because we're afraid to think of the bad or to hope for the good. Besides, it's the surprises that make the best plot twists. My life is nothing like I imagined, and so much better than I could have expected, and that goes for this moment in my life, when I am beginning to flirt with the idea of old age. I have a feeling I may be cut out to be an old woman. I was a weird little girl and an odd teenager, a mixture of bravado and insecurity that, together, was like one of those vinegar-and-baking-soda volcanoes you made for science as a kid, explosive and unpredictable. I felt as though my personality was not fit for a normal life in the world; I was always slightly at sea. Today I'm on terra firma. Will it last?

The great hallmark of my life, my generation, my time, has been choice. We've been a wandering breed, we Americans straddling the twentieth and twenty-first centuries, changing jobs, changing homes, changing spouses, religions, political parties. We've had more options than any generation before us, to marry those of different races or religions, to marry those of our own sex, to not marry at all but live together without legal obligation or live without a lifelong partner. I don't think any of this ever occurred to a man like my grandfather, who lived all his life in the city in which he was born, who took a job and stuck with it, who expected his children to do the same. Obligation trumped choice for his generation; for my own it is the other way around. The ability to exercise all those choices, to be a police officer who becomes a lawyer or a firefighter who becomes a florist, to raise kids in the suburbs and then leave for the city or even another country, have all given us a sense that we decide what happens next. Sometimes, if we dig deep, the choices are limited, even illusory. But we hold fast to the notion just the same.

It's not only death that terrifies us when we think about passing through the decades that come next. Maybe it's not even mainly death. It's the diminution of choices. There is nothing, nothing that enrages me more than listening to people talk about having those ugly little conversations with their aged parents. "That house is just too much for them," one will say. "I had to tell her that she just can't live alone anymore," another will add. "He just can't take care of himself," says a third. And my back goes up like a Halloween cat as I think: The people you are discussing are adults. They can make their own decisions, and they've earned the right to do so.

I don't like the notion of the child becoming father to the man, or, more likely, mother to the woman, perhaps because I saw firsthand how distressed my mother was by the notion. One day it was decided that she was too ill to do what she had always done, to be who she had always been, to put the chicken in the oven, to change the beds. When I showed up, with bad grace and humor, to take over her life, it must have seemed as though she was diminished, defeated, perhaps already dead.

On a sailing trip to the British Virgin Islands, the five of us, my husband and I and our three children, decided to swim from the dinghy to the rocky beach in a particularly vicious chop. I floundered in the strong current despite all my aerobic exercise and weight training and had to be helped to shore by the first mate, a lively college graduate who had been raised in St. Thomas and knew how to negotiate the undertow. "Charlotte saved my life!" I repeated jauntily during the rest of the trip, but at the time I didn't feel the least bit jaunty, simply aged and defeated and, yes, frightened—not frightened of death but of weakness and incapacity. Of course, I also had to swim back to the dinghy in the opposite direction, this time with a new sense of purpose, a sense that I would make it to that boat if it was the last thing I did. As I beat at the roiling sea with my oscillating arms, I heard one of my sons say in a panicky voice, "You okay, Mom?" And I am ashamed to admit that I shouted fiercely, "Leave me alone!" I apologized afterward for my overwrought response to his question, but I wasn't responding to his question at all. I was responding to my own fear, of burdening my children with concern, oversight, the need to take care of me, to someday decide that my home was too large or my stairs too steep. I was imagining what, for me, is the worst-case future.

When I think of that future, I know that my choices will narrow, have been narrowing as surely as a perspective drawing leading the eye to the focal point. I won't be going to medical school and becoming a surgeon. I'm not going to live in Italy or learn Chinese. I may have to become more thrifty and less spontaneous, may be lonelier and needier than I'd like. "Aging, particularly in the later decades, is a drawing in," Carolyn Heilbrun wrote when she herself was in her seventies. And I like drawing in okay. I like sitting in a big chair with a long book. I like spending an hour pulling together ingredients for a stew and then staying inside all day while its aroma seeps into every corner of the house. And later on, I don't mind dishing out a portion for myself alone and eating it while I read, my book to one side of the plate, although I prefer dishing it out to my husband and our children and listening to them all talk together, like a tennis match of words and jokes and old, old stories.

I think I could be okay with that more solitary life. But I would like to be strong and healthy enough to control how I live it. Each summer I go to the cemetery and lay a few flowers on the grave of a woman named Maxine Smiley, who was once our next-door neighbor. She was in her seventies when we first met her, and she and my toddler daughter struck up an unlikely friendship abetted by a break in the hedge between our properties and the fact that they were two of the most strong-minded

people I have ever met. Maria would light Mrs. Smiley's cigarette; once, when she began to give her the enlightened modern
child's view of smoking, acquired in a school session on good
health, Mrs. Smiley said, "If you do that you can't come here
anymore." Sometimes I would see Maria stalk across our lawn,
the out-thrust bottom lip visible despite the lowered head, and
when she got to the door she would mutter, "Mrs. Smiley was
crabby to me," and go off to find her brothers. But when she had
to write an essay in sixth grade about a person who had made a
difference in her life, she wrote about Mrs. Smiley and titled it
"My Best Friend."

I, too, cut through the hedge to visit Mrs. Smiley, trading
local gossip and updates on the state of the produce available at
the farm stands in the area, the sweet corn, the white peaches. I
admired the fact that she always cooked for herself, ate dinner
on a tray table when she was alone but always ate well, a nice
salad, broiled fish with a dill or caper sauce. I never stayed too
long when I went to see her because it was clear that Mrs. Smiley welcomed visitors, and welcomed their leave-taking as well.
She read, watched certain TV programs, spoke on the phone,
went to the market until she concluded that she ought no longer
to drive her big old sedan. "Other people want to go a lot faster
than I do," she said philosophically.

Every summer we would go out to dinner together, just the
two of us. It's the only time I've ever reserved a table in the
smoking section. I would never have told Mrs. Smiley what to
do, and neither, from my experience, would anyone else. And
perhaps as a result of that strength and specificity she had what
I think of as a good old age, in her own home, on her own schedule, by her own lights. She had one of those stupid accidents we
all sometimes have, the ones that become increasingly onerous
the older we become, and she wound up in the hospital for a
brief stay that ended in her death. But she didn't dwindle into
senescence or live in a place where she would have been con-

fined by four unfamiliar institutional walls, or, worse for a woman of her character, live surrounded by those she thought foolish and boring.

At dinner we would sometimes talk about the long span of her life. She'd been trained as a nurse but worked as one of the earliest flight attendants. The planes flew low, the trips were rocky, some of the passengers got sick. She raised an eyebrow whenever I mentioned the discomforts of modern flying, remembering those early days. She'd been born in one century and died in another. There was so much to remember, to amaze.

Anyone who was born, as I was, in the middle of the twentieth century and is now living through the early decades of the twenty-first should appreciate the feeling. What a time we've lived through, so revolutionary that the list could go on and on: the Pill, the heart transplant, the moon landings, cellphones, cable television, computer communication. As a small child I listened to the sound track of *South Pacific* on a series of long-playing albums; now I have it downloaded onto my laptop. When my boys were little and I worked at home I had one of the earliest personal computers, an IBM XT that made a sound like a stomach growling when it saved my documents. It had less memory than a digital watch does today.

On the morning after the presidential election of 2008, my father said, a catch in his voice, "I'm glad I've lived long enough to see the Phillies win the World Series and a black man elected president." I remember once sitting outside with Mrs. Smiley as an enormous jet passed silently overhead, like a shining exclamation point in the blue sky, and saying to her, remembering her stories of planes with no pressure and enough seats for only a handful of passengers, "That must be so strange for you."

"It's interesting," she'd replied, looking up.

I want to see what happens next. I want to see the future and be a little bit of a crank about the past, to tell my grandchildren stories about black-and-white televisions and cars without seatbelts and watch them light up when they're young and turn off when they're teenagers. I want to bore them with my memories, or what's left of them. People like to rehearse their worst fears by looking at them from a safe distance, denatured. In my case I've watched on more than a few occasions a lovely small movie called *Iris*. It's about the brilliant British writer Iris Murdoch, who wrote more than two dozen books and who was selected as one of the most influential English authors of the twentieth century. The film crosscuts between Murdoch's early years and her last ones, when she was locked in the dungeon of Alzheimer's. And no matter how often I've seen it, there is one moment when I always go over an emotional cliff. The actress Judi Dench, who plays Murdoch, turns to her husband and says, haltingly, as though she is pulling something precious from a deep dark pit, "I . . . wrote . . . books."

I want to be able to remember it all, not just the books but the newsrooms and the playgroups and the bad jokes and the holiday traditions. In my mind I can walk through the house where I grew up even though I have not been inside it for decades. (I did drive by once, a few years ago, sure that it would look shabby, diminished, not what I recalled. It looked exactly the same, foursquare and lovely.) I want to be able to walk through the house of my own life until my life is done. I want to hold on to who and what I have been even as both become somehow inevitably less.

Most of us convince ourselves that we will reach a plateau from our peak, not a valley. When we're young we take chances— we won't be the one who gets pregnant having unprotected sex or gets thrown from the speeding car when not belted in. Even as we become more responsible and wise, our mind tells us that we will beat the odds, that the mammogram and the colonoscopy are simply annoyances, to be gotten overwith.

And I suspect many of us feel the same way about advanced age. We visit a nursing home and see patients in the hallways, in wheelchairs, curved into themselves like invertebrates or staring blankly into the fuggy air. We hear of those whose minds have been wiped clean or whose bodies have become crippled. Or we simply have friends and relations dealing with the less important but still irritating inconveniences, the memory glitches, the incontinence, the falls. "If you break a hip, you're finished," Mrs. Smiley once told me. It was an overstatement, but I think what she was really trying to say was that sometimes a single moment can mark the dividing line between who you are and who you never wanted to be.

I try to imagine all the contingencies, but I admit I focus on the ones I like best. Sitting at a book club meeting next to a ninety-one-year-old woman, listening to her talk about taking the bus because cabs are highway robbery. Or hearing the story of a ninety-nine-year-old still practicing law. Or watching a woman who I'm certain is in her eighties whizzing by beneath the West Side Highway on in-line skates. Never mind that I have never been able to skate. Yes, yes, yes, I say to myself.

Occasionally, when I sit in the Adirondack chairs by the pond, I wonder if someday I will look down at my pants and shirt, my speckled arms and gnarled hands, and realize that I have finally become that woman I imagined I saw here one day long ago. Here is what I hope: I hope that woman does have grandchildren, and that they like to visit her, if only to see the snapping turtles in the pond or the Alice in Wonderland statue in Central Park. I hope her husband is still alive, and most of her friends, and please God her children, because there are some things she truly cannot bear. I hope she writes as often as she cares to, and that there are still readers who resonate to her words. I hope she can walk with pleasure and ease to the end of the long drive and back to get the mail from the box, stroll through Central Park to the museum and home again. I hope she has a good life, with just enough company. I hope, after breathing and swearing and sweating and wailing through three natural births, that she manages to have a natural death, without hospital rooms and fluorescent lighting and beeping machines. From her bedroom in the city she can hear the hum of raucous life in the streets outside; from her bedroom in the country she can see a long stretch of lawn and the occasional deer grazing at daybreak. Either bed would be a fine place to die when the time arrives.

But that time is not yet. For now, either bed is a fine place from which to start the day: power walk, newspapers, friends on the phone, words on the page, dinner with Gerry, Quin, Chris, and Maria. I couldn't imagine what it would be like, this growing older. I couldn't have imagined it would be like this. And so I say, and pray, and think again: To be continued. It's another day, and I'm off and running. See you.

ABOUT THE TYPE

This book was set in Granjon, a modern recutting of a typeface produced under the direction of George W. Jones, who based Granjon's design upon the letter forms of Claude Garamond (1480–1561). The name was given to the typeface as a tribute to the typographic designer Robert Granjon.

ANNA QUINDLEN

Every Last One

'Engrossing ... spellbinding'
NEW YORK TIMES

The Lathams seem to have it all: health, wealth and a vibrant family life. As Mary Beth Latham contemplates a life built around home, friends and community, she has every reason to feel fulfilled and content.

Then, for one of her sons, a process of unravelling begins. Mary Beth starts to focus on him, only to find that the comfortable life she has spent years carefully constructing is shattered in a single moment. Forced to confront her own demons, Mary Beth realises how the inconsequential moments we all share – and one shameful act she has hidden from everybody – may have contributed to her fate.

Every Last One is a mesmerising and devastating portrait of family life, and a testament to the power of a mother's love and determination. It is Anna Quindlen's finest work to date.

'A breathtaking novel. Quindlen writes superbly about families, grief and betrayal. I was completely mesmerised by this book and Mary Beth and the Latham family will stay with me for a long time to come'
LISA JEWELL

'Moves, in the turn of a page, from cosy, slow-burning American pastoral to the gripping stuff of nightmares'
GUARDIAN

ANNA QUINDLEN

Rise and Shine

It's an ordinary Monday morning when Meghan Fitzmaurice's perfect life implodes.

A household name as the host of talk show *Rise and Shine*, Meghan cuts to a commercial break, but not before she mutters two forbidden words into her open microphone.

In an instant, it's the end of an era, not only for Meghan, but also for her younger sister, Bridget, a social worker in the Bronx who has always lived in Meghan's long shadow. The effect of Meghan's on-air slip reverberates through the lives of everyone they know, and the sisters are forced to adapt and survive by using their quick wits and powerful connection, one that even the worst tragedy cannot shatter.

ANNA QUINDLEN

Blessings

One night a young couple sneak onto the estate of wealthy dowager Lydia Blessing and leave a box in the driveway. In the box is a newborn baby, and for Skip Cuddy, the caretaker who finds her, it is the discovery of a lifetime. In secret, he takes the baby in, and starts to care for her.

When Lydia uncovers the truth, she has choices to make, as she had many years before.

'We are so lucky to have Anna Quindlen in our literary lives. With her big heart and her amazing humanity she reminds us all of our blessings.'
ALICE HOFFMAN

'Qualities and shades of love are this writer's strong suit, and she has the unusual talent for writing about them with so much truth and heart that one is carried away on a tidal wave of involvement and concern.'
ELIZABETH JANE HOWARD

'Quindlen writes with power and grace.'
THE BOSTON GLOBE

ANNA QUINDLEN

Black and Blue

The first time my husband hit me I was nineteen years old

For eighteen years Fran Benedetto kept her secret, hid her bruises. She stayed with Bobby because she wanted her son to have a father, and because, in spite of everything, she loved him. Then one night, when she saw the look on her ten-year-old son's face, Fran finally made a choice – she ran for both their lives.

Now she is starting over in a city far from home, far from Bobby. She uses a name that isn't hers, watches over her son, and tries to forget. For the woman who now calls herself Beth, every day is a chance to heal, to put together the pieces of her shattered self. But every day she waits for Bobby to catch up to her. Bobby always said he would never let her go, and Fran Benedetto is certain of one thing: It is only a matter of time.

'The honesty of her storytelling is exemplary'
SUNDAY TELEGRAPH

'Quindlen has got so deeply inside her characters that they gave me nightmares'
THE TIMES

'Quindlen proves herself a virtuoso . . . vivid, compassionate and tense'
THE NEW YORK TIMES

ANNA QUINDLEN

One True Thing

'Simply impossible to forget'
ALICE HOFFMAN

Ellen Gulden is a successful, young New York journalist. But
when her mother, Kate, is diagnosed with cancer, she leaves
her life in the city to return home and care for her. In the short
time they have left, the relationship between mother and
daughter – tender, awkward and revealing – deepens, and Ellen
is forced to confront painful truths about her adored father.

But in the weeks that follow Kate's death, events take a shocking and unexpected turn. Family emotions are laid bare as a
new drama is played out, and overnight Ellen goes from
devoted daughter to prime suspect, accused of the mercy
killing of her 'one true thing'.

One True Thing is the devastating story of a mother and daughter,
of love and loss, and of shattering choices.

'The relationship between mother and daughter is a triumph.
This novel deserves to be bought, read and kept'
ELIZABETH JANE HOWARD

'Quindlen's extraordinarily moving novel is about responsibilities,
compassion and growing up'
DAILY MAIL

ANNA QUINDLEN

Object Lessons

It is the 1960s, in suburban New York City, and twelve-year-old Maggie Scanlan begins to sense that beneath the calm surface of her peaceful life, things are going strangely wrong.

When her all-powerful grandfather is struck down by a stroke, the reverberations affect Maggie's entire family. Her normally dispassionate father breaks down, her mother becomes distant and unavailable, and matters only get worse when her cousin and her best friend start doing things to each other that leave Maggie confused about sex and terrified of sin. With all of this upheaval how can she be sure that what she wants is even worth having?

'Quindlen is at her best writing about the dislocations of growing up, the blows a child does not see coming'
TIME

'Elaborate and playful ...Honest and deeply felt ...Here is the Quindlen wit, the sharp eye for the details of class and manners, [and] the ardent reading of domestic lives'
THE NEW YORK TIMES